FOGSI EEBR 2025
Ethical Evidence-Based Recommendations
Postpartum Hemorrhage

Disclaimer

This Ethical Evidence-Based Recommendation (EEBR) document is drafted following a consensus between esteemed FOGSI experts and stakeholders and are based on the scientific evidence available at the time of preparation.

EEBRs should be used for information and educational purposes. They do not replace the need for application of clinical judgment to each individual presentation, or variations based on individual patient and resource setting.

Furthermore, EEBRs do not constitute or imply the endorsement of any of the included technologies, therapies, or techniques by FOGSI.

FOGSI EEBR 2025
Ethical Evidence-Based Recommendations
Postpartum Hemorrhage

Editor-in-Chief

Sunita Tandulwadkar
MD (Obs and Gyne) FICS (Gyne-Endoscopy) FICOG
President, FOGSI (2025–2026)
Gynecological Endoscopist and ART & IVF Specialist
Head, Department of Obstetrics and Gynecology
Chief, IVF & Endoscopy Center, Ruby Hall Clinic, Pune
Founder and Medical Director
Solo Clinic IVF—A Center for Excellence in Infertility and Endoscopy, Pune
Founder and Medical Director
Solo Stem Cells—A Stem Cell Research and Application Center, Pune
Founder and Director, Alive Regenerative Wellness, Pune, Maharashtra, India

Editors

Sheela Mane
MD FRCOG FICOG FICMCH
Consultant
Anugraha Nursing Home, Bengaluru
Professor
Department Obstetrics and Gynecology
DNB Faculty
KC General Hospital
Bengaluru, Karnataka, India
Vice Chair, ICOG 2024

Sushil Chawla
MS DNB MNAMS FICOG FAIMER Fellowship
Professor and Head
Department Obstetrics and Gynecology
INHS Asvini
Mumbai, Maharashtra, India

Experts

Mahesh Gupta
MD (Gynec)
High Risk Pregnancy Expert
Pushpam and Matis Multispeciality Hospital,
Tertiary Referral Centre for Placenta
Acreta Spectrum
Ahmedabad, Gujarat, India

Manish R Pandya
MD FICOG FICMH PhD
Professor and Head
Department of Obstetrics and Gynecology
Mahavir Hospital and Manish IVF Center
Surendranagar, Gujarat, India

Convener

Pooja Lodha
DNB (Obs and Gyne)
Fellow, Fetal Medicine, FOGSI-FMF UK Certified
Lead Consultant
Department of Fetal Medicine
Ruby Hall Clinic and Bharati Vidyapeeth University and Hospital, Pune
Director, Kangaroo Cradle, Fetal Care Centre
Pune, Maharashtra, India

JAYPEE BROTHERS MEDICAL PUBLISHERS
The Health Sciences Publisher
New Delhi | London

Jaypee Brothers Medical Publishers (P) Ltd

Headquarters
Jaypee Brothers Medical Publishers (P) Ltd
EMCA House, 23/23-B
Ansari Road, Daryaganj
New Delhi 110 002, India
Landline: +91-11-23272143, +91-11-23272703
+91-11-23282021, +91-11-23245672
Email: jaypee@jaypeebrothers.com

Corporate Office
Jaypee Brothers Medical Publishers (P) Ltd
4838/24, Ansari Road, Daryaganj
New Delhi 110 002, India
Phone: +91-11-43574357
Fax: +91-11-43574314
Email: jaypee@jaypeebrothers.com

Overseas Office
JP Medical Ltd.
83, Victoria Street, London
SW1H 0HW (UK)
Phone: +44 20 3170 8910
Fax: +44 (0)20 3008 6180
Email: info@jpmedpub.com

Website: www.jaypeebrothers.com
Website: www.jaypeedigital.com

Inquiries for bulk sales may be solicited at: jaypee@jaypeebrothers.com

FOGSI EEBR 2025—Ethical Evidence-Based Recommendations: Postpartum Hemorrhage

First Edition: **2025**

ISBN: 978-93-6616-756-5

Printed in India

Contributors

Ashis K Mukhopadhyay
MBBS DGO DNBOG FICOG
Professor, Unit Chief and Principal
Department Obstetrics and Gynecology
CSS College of Obstetrics, Gynecology and Child Health
Kolkata, West Bengal, India

BS Susheela Rani
MD PGDMLE FICOG
Medical Director and Consultant
Department Obstetrics and Gynecology
Manjushree Speciality Hospital
Bengaluru, Karnataka, India

Gowri Sayiprasad
MBBS MS DNB FMAS
Professor and Unit Head
Department Obstetrics and Gynecology
Prakash Institute of Medical Sciences
Islampur, Maharashtra, India

Haresh Doshi
MD (Gynec) PhD FICOG Diploma (USG) PGDMLS PGDCR PGCML PGDHHM
Professor and Head
Department of Obstetrics and Gynecology
GCS Medical College, Hospital and Research Center
Ahmedabad, Gujarat, India

Latha Venkataram
FRCOG (UK) MRCP(I)
Director, WMN Healthcare Services Pvt Ltd, Bengaluru
Lead Consultant
Department of Obstetrics and Gynecology
Rangadore Memorial Hospital
Bengaluru, Karnataka, India
President, Bangalore RCOG Trust

Madhva Prasad
MS DNB PGDMLS PGDCR ACME
Associate Professor
Department Obstetrics and Gynecology
St John's Medical College
Bengaluru, Karnataka, India

Mahesh Gupta
MD (Gynec)
High Risk Pregnancy Expert
Pushpam and Matis Multispeciality Hospital, Tertiary Referral Centre for Placenta Acreta Spectrum
Ahmedabad, Gujarat, India

Manish R Pandya
MD FICOG FICMH PhD
Professor and Head
Department of Obstetrics and Gynecology
Mahavir Hospital and Manish IVF Center
Surendranagar, Gujarat, India

Mousumi Das Ghosh
MD FICOG
Senior Consultant and Unit Head
Department Obstetrics and Gynecology
Tata Main Hospital and Manipal Tata Medical College
Jamshedpur, Jharkhand, India

Mrutyunjaya Bellad
MD (Obs and Gyne) FICOG
Professor
Department of Obstetrics and Gynecology
KAHER's JN Medical College
Belagavi, Karnataka, India

Nalini Mishra
MD DNB FICOG MNAMS
Dean and Professor
Department Obstetrics and Gynecology
LN Medical College and Research Centre
Bhopal, Madhya Pradesh, India

Pooja Patil
MS (Obs and Gyne) MRCOG FICOG FMAS
Professor and Head
Department of Obstetrics and Gynecology
LN Medical College
Bhopal, Madhya Pradesh, India

Poonam Varma Shivkumar
MS
Director–Professor
Department of Obstetrics and Gynecology
Unit Chief and Medical Superintendent
Mahatma Gandhi Institute of Medical Sciences
Wardha, Maharashtra, India

Rajesh Sharma
MS (Obs and Gyne) ART
Head
Department of Obstetrics and Gynecology
151 Base Hospital
Guwahati, Assam, India

Sadhana Gupta
MS (Gold Medalist) MNAMS FICOG FIUMB FICMCH
Director and Senior Consultant
Department of Obstetrics and Gynecology
Jeevan Jyoti Hospital and Medical Research Centre
Gorakhpur, Uttar Pradesh, India
Vice Chair-Elect, ICOG 2025

Saswati Sanyal Choudhury
MD FICOG FICMCH FIAOG
Professor
Department of Obstetrics and Gynecology
Gauhati Medical College
Guwahati, Assam, India

Seema Mehrotra
MBBS MS
Professor
Department Obstetrics and Gynecology
King George's Medical University
Lucknow, Uttar Pradesh, India

Shalini Gainder
MD FICOG FMAS
Professor
Department of Obstetrics and Gynecology
Postgraduate Institute of Medical Education and Research
Chandigarh, India

Shashi L Kabra Maheshwari
MD FICOG FMAS DIPMAS
Senior Specialist
Department Obstetrics and Gynecology
DDU Hospital
New Delhi, India

Sheela Mane
MD FRCOG FICOG FICMCH
Consultant
Anugraha Nursing Home, Bengaluru
Professor
Department Obstetrics and Gynecology
DNB Faculty
KC General Hospital
Bengaluru, Karnataka, India
Vice Chair, ICOG 2024

Shikha Seth
MD FICS FICOG
Professor and Head
Department Obstetrics and Gynecology
All India Institute of Medical Sciences
Gorakhpur, Uttar Pradesh, India

Srimathy Raman
MD FRCOG CCT (UK)
Consultant
Department Obstetrics and Gynecology
Rangadore Memorial Hospital
Bengaluru, Karnataka, India

Sunita Tandulwadkar
MD (Obs and Gyne) FICS (Gyne-Endoscopy) FICOG
President, FOGSI (2025–2026)
Gynecological Endoscopist and ART & IVF Specialist
Head, Department of Obstetrics and Gynecology
Chief, IVF & Endoscopy Center
Ruby Hall Clinic, Pune
Founder and Medical Director
Solo Clinic IVF—A Center for Excellence in Infertility and Endoscopy, Pune
Founder and Medical Director
Solo Stem Cells—A Stem Cell Research and Application Center, Pune
Founder and Director
Alive Regenerative Wellness
Pune, Maharashtra, India

Sushil Chawla
MS DNB MNAMS FICOG FAIMER Fellowship
Professor and Head
Department Obstetrics and Gynecology
INHS Asvini
Mumbai, Maharashtra, India

T Chitra
MD (Obs and Gyne) DNB MNAMS
Fellowship in RM and Laparoscopy
Professor
Department Obstetrics and Gynecology
Jawaharlal Institute of Postgraduate Medical Education and Research
Puducherry, India

Vidyadhar Bangal
MD DNB MPH PhD
Professor and Head
Department Obstetrics and Gynecology
Pravara Institute of Medical Sciences
Ahmednagar, Maharashtra, India

Executive Summary

"Quickly grasp the key elements and novel insights of our leading-edge recommendations."

Postpartum hemorrhage (PPH) remains a significant cause of maternal morbidity and mortality worldwide. A panel of experts across India has developed modified and adoptable recommendations for the management of PPH, focusing on evidence and innovative approaches. Emphasis is placed on a multidisciplinary approach, continuous patient monitoring, and regular updates. Key recommendations include the use of uterotonics for prevention, early identification of high-risk patients, implementation of nonsurgical interventions like balloon tamponade, and timely surgical measures when necessary. This comprehensive approach encompasses every stage of PPH management, from risk identification to post-treatment care, and is meticulously grounded in the latest scientific research and clinical best practices. Designed to be universally applicable, these recommendations cater to a diverse array of healthcare settings, including high-resource hospitals and low-resource community clinics.

On a national level, the implementation of these recommendations aims to standardize PPH management practices, ensuring consistency in care and delivery across different regions and healthcare facilities. By adopting these recommendations, we anticipate a substantial reduction in both the incidence and the severity of PPH, thereby significantly enhancing maternal health outcomes across the country. Furthermore, these recommendations serve as a foundation for developing national policies and protocols that can be tailored to the specific needs and resources of individual regions, promoting equitable and effective PPH management nationwide.

Preface

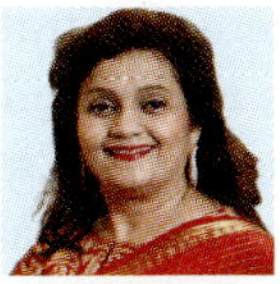

Editor-in-Chief
Sunita Tandulwadkar

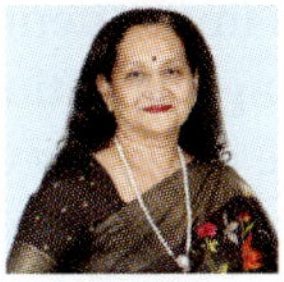

Editor
Sheela Mane

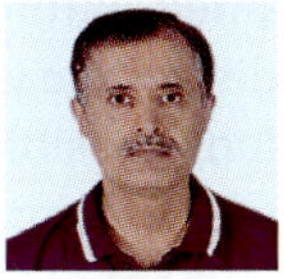

Editor
Sushil Chawla

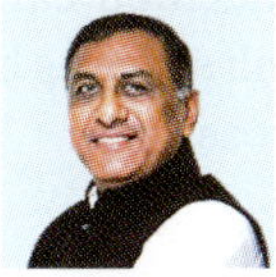

Expert
Mahesh Gupta

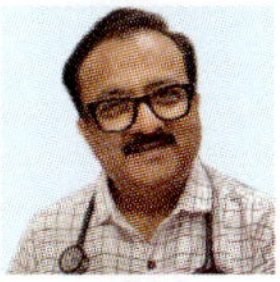

Expert
Manish R Pandya

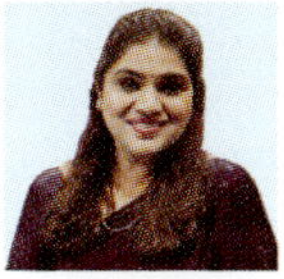

Convener
Pooja Lodha

In our pursuit of advancing women's health in India, establishing our own ethical evidence-based recommendations is essential. As the President of the Federation of Obstetric and Gynaecological Societies of India (FOGSI) 2025, I am delighted to present this *Ethical Evidence-Based Recommendations on Postpartum Hemorrhage*, a comprehensive resource developed through the collaborative expertise of leading professionals across the country. While international organizations such as the International Federation of Gynecology and Obstetrics (FIGO), American Society for Reproductive Medicine (ASRM), European Society of Human Reproduction and Embryology (ESHRE), and Royal College of Obstetricians and Gynaecologists (RCOG) have established extensive recommendations, India has yet to provide a cohesive, evidence-backed framework tailored for postpartum hemorrhage. This publication bridges that gap, equipping Indian practitioners with practical, scientifically grounded recommendations for managing postpartum hemorrhage (PPH) in diverse clinical settings.

Postpartum hemorrhage remains one of the most significant challenges in obstetrics, with potential implications for maternal morbidity and mortality. These ethical evidence-based recommendations begin with definitions and terminologies, providing a foundational understanding of PPH classifications. Early risk identification follows, outlining protocols to detect women at higher risk of PPH, allowing for pre-emptive measures to reduce incidence and improve outcomes.

The publication then addresses preventive strategies, offering evidence-backed approaches to minimizing the likelihood of PPH. A comprehensive section on medical management explores pharmaceutical options for controlling hemorrhage, while hemo-resuscitation guidelines ensure that practitioners can respond swiftly to blood loss with life-saving interventions. Recommendations for minimal surgical management are presented, alongside more advanced surgical interventions to equip practitioners with a range of options, depending on the severity and nature of the hemorrhage.

A dedicated section on traumatic PPH covers management strategies for cases resulting from trauma, while secondary PPH is addressed with protocols for identifying and managing delayed hemorrhage cases. Special situations are also discussed, offering guidance for complex cases that may fall outside standard PPH protocols.

The recommendations include practical tools and resources designed to support effective PPH management, as well as a section on implementation and training, recognizing that skilled execution and ongoing education are key to improving outcomes. A summary provides a concise overview of the key points, enabling practitioners to quickly review essential practices and recommendations.

This publication represents FOGSI's commitment to equipping Indian gynecologists with the latest scientific advancements, framed within our cultural and clinical context. I am deeply grateful to the multidisciplinary team whose collaborative efforts have made these recommendations possible. We hope they become a trusted companion for practitioners, empowering them to deliver compassionate, evidence-based care in the management of PPH.

Through this initiative, FOGSI reaffirms its dedication to advancing women's health and setting a new standard for ethical, informed care. We trust that these ethical evidence-based recommendations will serve as both a valuable guide and an inspiration for PPH management across India.

Preface

It is with great pride and satisfaction that we present this *Ethical Evidence-Based Recommendations on Postpartum Hemorrhage*. This book is the culmination of years of dedicated research, clinical experience, and a shared passion for improving maternal health.

Postpartum hemorrhage (PPH) remains a significant global health challenge, claiming countless lives each year. Despite advancements in medical science, this preventable condition continues to pose a serious threat to maternal mortality and morbidity. This book aims to address this pressing issue by providing up-to-date information, evidence-based guidelines, and practical strategies for the prevention, diagnosis, and management of PPH.

Our goal is to empower healthcare providers worldwide with the knowledge and tools necessary to effectively address PPH. This book covers a wide range of topics, including epidemiology, risk factors, pathophysiology, clinical presentation, and diagnostic evaluation of PPH. It also delves into the latest advancements in medical and surgical interventions, as well as nonpharmacological approaches.

We have meticulously reviewed the latest research and clinical guidelines to ensure that the information presented in this book is accurate, relevant, and evidence based. We have also incorporated real-world experiences and insights from our own clinical practice to provide practical guidance for healthcare providers at all levels.

We extend our sincere gratitude to all the experts (Dr Mahesh Gupta, Dr Manish Pandya), colleagues, and institutions who have contributed to this endeavor. Their support and guidance have been invaluable in shaping this book. We also acknowledge the tireless efforts of our dedicated team, who worked diligently to bring this book to fruition. Our special thanks to Dr Sunita Tandulwadkar for this initiative and Dr Pooja Lodha for keeping us on our toes.

We hope that this book will serve as a valuable resource for healthcare providers, researchers, and students alike. By improving our understanding and management of PPH, we can work towards a future where every woman can experience a safe and healthy childbirth.

Sheela Mane
Sushil Chawla

Contents

CHAPTER 1

Introduction

Sheela Mane

"Dive into the essentials of effective postpartum hemorrhage management."

Postpartum hemorrhage (PPH) is a significant global maternal health challenge. Effective management of PPH is crucial due to its significant impact on maternal health. PPH remains a leading cause of maternal morbidity and mortality. Timely and appropriate management is essential to prevent severe complications and save lives. These recommendations emphasize the importance of evidence-based practices and innovative approaches to improve the detection, prevention, and treatment of PPH.

Standardization of PPH definitions and diagnostic criteria is essential for accurate clinical assessment and data comparison. Early identification and management are crucial for improving outcomes. Risk factor assessment is important for targeted prevention, but it is essential to recognize that PPH can occur without identifiable risk factors.

This document covers a wide range of topics including defining PPH, identifying risk factors, and implementing prevention strategies. Medical and surgical management options, including the use of blood products, are detailed. Special considerations for traumatic PPH, secondary PPH, and specific patient populations are addressed. Additionally, the document outlines essential tools, resources, and training for healthcare providers to effectively manage PPH. Addressing challenges in low-resource settings and leveraging technology are crucial for improving PPH outcomes globally.

The primary purpose of these recommendations is to offer healthcare professionals a clear and concise framework for the effective management of postpartum hemorrhage (PPH). By standardizing care protocols, these recommendations aim to enhance the quality of care, reduce variability in treatment approaches, and improve overall maternal outcomes. These recommendations are designed for a wide range of healthcare professionals, including obstetricians, midwives, nurses, anesthetists, and emergency medical personnel. They are applicable across diverse healthcare settings, from high-resource hospitals to low-resource community clinics, ensuring that all providers have access to best practices for managing PPH.

The recommendations delineate the roles and responsibilities of healthcare teams in managing PPH, which include maintaining accurate and thorough documentation of all PPH-related incidents and interventions, conducting regular training drills to ensure team preparedness and effective response to PPH events, and following standardized protocols to ensure a cohesive and efficient approach to PPH management. By adhering to these recommendations, healthcare professionals can significantly improve maternal outcomes through standardized, evidence-based management of postpartum hemorrhage. This comprehensive approach ensures that healthcare providers are equipped with the necessary tools and knowledge to effectively address PPH in various clinical settings.

By addressing these critical aspects, the introduction sets the stage for the comprehensive and detailed guidance provided in the subsequent sections of the document, ensuring that all healthcare providers are well-equipped to manage PPH effectively. This document outlines key aspects of PPH prevention, management, and training.

CHAPTER 2

Background of Postpartum Hemorrhage

Madhva Prasad

BACKGROUND

"To understand the global challenge of PPH and the journey to these recommendations."

- **Briefing:**
  - Global and regional epidemiology of postpartum hemorrhage (PPH)
  - Review of latest FIGO/WHO recommendations
  - Recent advances in PPH research
- **Unanswered Questions:**
  - What factors drive the epidemiology and outcomes of the problem?
  - How has the integration of previous recommendations impacted the standard of care and outcomes in various healthcare settings?
  - How reliable are the recommendations being suggested?
- **Recommendations**

Q1. Global and regional epidemiology of PPH.

Draft recommendations: There is wide variation in the prevalence of PPH across the word (1–10%), with notable differences between different regions. The estimated occurrence of PPH appears to have increased in the recent decades. The contribution of PPH to mortality, near-miss events, and morbidity is significant.

Discussion/review of literature: Postpartum hemorrhage (PPH) complicates around 1–10% of all births. Approximately 80,000 maternal deaths worldwide were attributable to PPH in the year 2015. Due to variations in definition and reporting of PPH, the "FIGO PPH 2022" document acknowledges that pinpointing a prevalence rate of PPH is a major challenge. In an earlier systematic review, Carroli et al. pegged the prevalence of PPH to be around 6% and severe PPH to be around 1.86% of all deliveries, with a wide variation across the world. The respective regional prevalence of PPH was calculated in Africa to be 10.45%, Australasia 7.68% Latin America 8.90%, North America/ Europe 6.3%, and Asia 2.55%. The respective regional prevalence of severe PPH was calculated in Africa to be 2.21%, Asia 1.78%, Europe 1.75%, Latin America 5.3%, and Australasia 4.3%. Though Asians appear to have a lesser propensity for PPH, there seems to be higher occurrence of severe PPH, probably due to disparities in access to medical care. In a subsequent analysis, Calvert et al. (2012) suggest that PPH (when defined as blood loss more than 500 mL) has been reported to range from 7% in developed countries, all the way up to 25% in African countries. When defined as blood loss more than 1000 mL, it has been reported to range from 5.1% in African countries and 1.9% in Asian countries.

However, the occurrence of PPH was either underestimated before, or has increased recently. Recent review articles (2022) suggest the pooled prevalence of PPH in Ethiopia only is estimated to be 11.4%. Similarly, recent Asian estimates are ranged around 17% for postpartum hemorrhage and 6% for severe PPH. Also, the impact of the problem is quite high**.** In the sub-Saharan African region alone, this case fatality rate ranges between 2.8 and 27.3%. World over too, the case fatality rate (or mortality index) for PPH is quite high 6.6% (ranging from 0 to 40%). The occurrence of near-miss cases is also significant (3 per 1,000 live births).

Q2. Recent guidelines and updates

Draft recommendations: Clinicians must acknowledge the presence of a vast variety of guidelines and documents which are regularly updated regarding the topic of PPH and must attempt to update themselves regularly. These must be adapted to clinicians' local situations and needs.

Discussion: Clinicians must acknowledge that there are very many documents released in the recent past, which summarily cover various details regarding PPH and its management strategies. A recent landmark publication in this regard is the FIGO recommendations on the management of postpartum hemorrhage 2022. Publications by WHO and FOGSI are also of keen interest and importance. While a variety of recommendations and suggestions exist, few may work better than the others in each clinician's local contexts. Hence, they may be adapted suitably for clinicians' local situations and needs.

Q3. What are some recent advances in PPH research?

Draft recommendations: Clinicians must be aware of a large number of exciting research that is taking place in the arena of PPH, and attempt to incorporate these into their own practice.

Evidence summary:

- Research in PPH can be categorized into many entities.
- Genomic association suggesting a role for progesterone receptor variations
- A novel device for autotransfusion of blood in life-threatening postpartum hemorrhage has been described.

- Wearable digital postpartum hemorrhage management device has been described, which helps in early identification of the postpartum hemorrhage and its consequences.
- A novel physiological method of "Squatting out the placenta" has been described but not studied adequately.
- Administration of calcium to prevent uterine atony has not been studied adequately.
- Many pharmacological agents are being explored for prevention and treatment of PPH. Candidate drugs in the preclinical stage included an antiarrhythmic (dofetilide with nanoparticle delivery) and a beta-blocker (propranolol). Other candidate drugs include a uterotonic (heat-stable inhaled oxytocin) and a blood-related product (ethamsylate). Candidates in Phase II include a vascular agent (vasopressin) and an antioxidant (melatonin).
- Creation, validation, and utilization of comprehensive digital phenotypes could be utilized for tracking outcomes and ongoing clinical research to deliver better preventative interventions for postpartum hemorrhage.
- Novel methods like postpartum uterine ultrasonographic scale can help in numerical assessment of uterine involution and prediction of secondary PPH.
- Use of real-time intraoperative blood loss monitoring using novel tablet applications need further studies in cesarean sections.
- Use of real-time measurement of hemoglobin using novel techniques are being investigated.
- Pilot studies of an innovative digital health tool called "the AccuFlow sensor" has shown some effectiveness.

Q4. "What factors drive the epidemiology and outcomes of the problem?"

Draft recommendations: Postpartum hemorrhage is condition which is heavily influenced by the level of facility at which the delivery takes place, skill level of available health personnel, awareness of healthcare personnel regarding available medications and provision of systems for quality drugs like oxytocin. Systems strengthening is needed for effective implementation of guidelines at the point-of-care.

Summary/review of evidence: Despite the presence of so many recommendations and guideline statements, very many bottlenecks are present which prevent the effective implementation of standards to the delivering woman at the end-user's location. Ameh et al. reviewed from an implementation research point of view with respect to "unmet need of standard for PPH care". The factors that stood out were location of delivery, provision for review of patient by a medical practitioner, provision for review of patient by a trained specialist. This was supplanted by major concerns at the point-of-care regarding use of misoprostol by unskilled healthcare personnel, availability of drugs like misoprostol, tranexamic acid, carbetocin; healthcare personnel awareness about these drugs and cold chain maintained oxytocin.

Q5. How has the integration of previous recommendations impacted the standard of care and outcomes in various healthcare settings?

Draft recommendations: Deaths due to postpartum hemorrhage may be reducing, but the proportion of PPH cases where major interventions are being done may be increasing.

Discussion/review of literature: Considering the fact that PPH is one of the biggest contributors to maternal mortality, the rapid Indian strides in reduction of the MMR—value of 97 (95% CI of 88–106) for years 2018-2020, suggests that the recommendations have indeed percolated, when viewed from a macro-level. However, there is still a lot left to be achieved. Ahmadzia et al. looked into trends of proportion of PPH cases needing interventions. In a temporal comparison between two decades (2000s and 2010s), though the rate of non-severe PPH did not change much (25.2 vs. 24.2 per 1,000), the rate of PPH needing blood transfusion among cesarean deliveries showed increase (2 to 4.8). PPH needing other interventions (0.9 to 1.9), hysterectomy (0.5 to 0.7), uterine artery embolization (0.3 to 0.5), and uterine tamponade (0.09 to 0.69) (all p values <0.001) showed increase. Clinicians in India must acknowledge that before we achieve a reduction of impact of PPH, a brief trend of increase in major interventions for PPH may be expected.

Q6. How reliable are the guidelines being generated worldwide?

Draft recommendations: Clinicians must be aware that there may be some gaps between recommendations and actual performance of these recommendations due to difficulties in recruitment of patients in trials, who are perfectly comparable to real-world situations.

Discussion/evidence: Some discordance has been noted between the reported occurrence of PPH in real-life settings and controlled settings like trials. The rates observed in trials where interventions are performed does not correspond to the estimates of global prevalence of PPH given by WHO. Also, there is a tendency to not include patients with high-risks into trials involving interventions for PPH. A reasonably large selection bias may be in play. Some unexpected findings of lesser-than-expected frequency of PPH in high-risk women and higher-than-expected frequency of PPH in low-risk women have been noted and may be secondary to differential levels of vigilance and enhanced monitoring among the high-risk women.

Unanswered questions: Whether patients with complicated pregnancies respond to uterotonics in equivalence to low-risk patients is unanswered. How patients who develop PPH unpredictably can be recruited into trials is an unanswered question.

BIBLIOGRAPHY

1. Bischoff K, Nothacker M, Lehane C, et al. Lack of controlled studies investigating the risk of postpartum haemorrhage in cesarean delivery after prior use of oxytocin: a scoping review. BMC Pregnancy Childbirth. 2017;17(1):399.
2. Hawker L, Weeks A. Postpartum haemorrhage (PPH) rates in randomized trials of PPH prophylactic interventions and the effect of underlying participant PPH risk: a meta-analysis. BMC Pregnancy Childbirth. 2020;20(1):107.
3. Martins RIL, Novais JSM, Reis ZSN. Postpartum haemorrhage in electronic health records: risk factors at admission and in-hospital occurrence. Rev Bras Ginecol Obstet. 2024;46:e-rbgo14.
4. Xu C, Zhong W, Fu Q, et al. Differential effects of different delivery methods on progression to severe postpartum haemorrhage between Chinese nulliparous and multiparous women: a retrospective cohort study. BMC Pregnancy Childbirth. 2020;20(1):660.

3

CHAPTER

Definition and Terminology

Sadhana Gupta, Shikha Seth, Mousumi Das Ghosh, Pooja Patil

Q1. Why do we need standardized definition: a clinically measurable, reproducible and applicable definition for all resource settings for prompt diagnosis of postpartum hemorrhage (PPH)?

Draft recommendations: PPH definition and diagnostic criteria as well as severity grading based on hemodynamic assessment, i.e., change in common clinically measurable vital parameters (as pulse, blood pressure, respiratory rate, temperature, consciousness, and SpO_2) is better option as they cover the concealed hemorrhage and capacity of any woman's tolerance to blood loss instead of blood loss quantification.

Summary of evidence:

Q1.1. Why we need standardized definition?

Currently PPH definitions is not standardized. WHO, ACOG, RCOG, FOGSI, FIGO terminology, definition criteria and severity staging differ **(Table 1)**

TABLE 1: Definitions of acute PPH by various obstetric societies.

Guideline/year	***Definition of PPH***	***Remarks***
WHO 2022		
Latest FIGO and ICM 2022	Estimated blood loss of more than 500 mL within 24 hours of a vaginal birth or 1,000 mL after cesarean section, *or* Any blood loss sufficient to compromise hemodynamic stability	Definition has two criteria QBL and hemodynamic assessment
FOGSI: 2018	>500 mL blood loss regardless of route of delivery	Only loss quantification
RCOG 2016	>500 mL regardless of route of delivery • *Mild:* 500–1000 mL, • *Moderate:* 1000–2000 mL, • *Severe:* >2000 mL	Required quantification measures
ACOG 2017: Revised	Defines PPH as cumulative blood loss ≥1,000 mL or blood loss accompanied by signs or symptoms of hypovolemia within 24 hours after the birth process (including intrapartum) *regardless* of route of delivery	Improved definition after 2017 modification

Q1.2. PPH classification and terminology.

Terms like primary and secondary PPH along with severity grading standardization are a must for early identification and timely interventions. Primary PPH, acute PPH, early PPH: blood loss of at least 500 mL, from the genital tract within 24 hours of delivery more than 1000 ml in cesarean section. Secondary PPH, late PPH or delayed PPH excessive blood loss from 24 hours to 12 weeks after birth (RCOG) 6 weeks (FOGSI, FIGO)

Currently the severity grading is defined based on blood loss quantification or percentage of total body blood volume loss as follows, which is really difficult to quantify and standardized tools not available. Hence the use of quantified blood loss, use of clinical parameters is recommended to be used for assessing the severity of PPH.

Q1.3. Severity grading of PPH (Table 2)

TABLE 2: Severity grading of PPH.

Grading	***Blood loss***	***RCOG classification***	
Grade I	500–1,000 mL	Minor	
Grade II	1000–1,500 mL	Major	Moderate
Grade III	1,500–2,000 mL		Severe
Grade IV	>2,000 mL		Massive

Q2. Is it quantification of blood loss (QBL) or the clinical condition/findings which should be the criteria for the diagnosis of PPH?

Draft recommendations: Hemodynamic parameters based severity grading are a better option for early identification, planning management, switching the interventions or for the referral, as they are directly quantifiable and simple. Blood loss quantification by visual estimation is grossly inaccurate and not recommended while the actual quantification of blood loss (aQBL) is another option with standardized algorithm and tools.

Summary evidence:

Quantitative measurement of blood loss is feasible and most definitions suggest cumulative quantification of blood loss at time of delivery.

- Hypovolemia created by PPH can be equivalized with shock, therefore, obstetric shock indexing (OSI) is simple easy to calculate tool for assessing significant loss as it helps in early diagnosis and have implications in PPH management.
- Mean arterial pressure (MAP) is another surrogate for reduced blood volume.
- MEOWS is best to be followed as it defines the buffer and alert zones, color coded, and have clear cut-off values.

There is insufficient evidence to recommend QBL over clinical estimation of blood loss.

Once PPH is defined, it should be "staged/graded". There are two options:

1. Direct by quantification of blood loss (QBL)
2. Indirectly by Shock grading. (clinical shock indexing)

Commonly used hypovolemia and shock classification are Advanced Trauma Life Support (ATLS) and Modified Early Obstetric Warning Signs (MEOWS). Problem with ATLS classification is that it does not seem to reflect clinical reality accurately.

Q3. How to quantify the blood loss (QBL) standard criteria and tools workable at low resource settings?

Visual estimation of blood loss is highly subjective and imprecise and it underestimates the actual blood loss when volumes are high. Although some visual volume appreciation tools are defined in literature as percentage of soaked pad/mop/bedsheet, etc., but not much effective **(Fig. 1)**. Approximately 30% error possible with visual method compared with the gravimetric technique of scaling.

Q3.1. Actual quantification of blood loss (aQBL)

Gross blood loss is measured in a graduated containers as suction jars (in cesarean) and under buttock pouches (vaginal delivery) **(Fig. 2)**. All the soaked blood cloths, bed linen and mops weight are measured on scale and their dry weight is subtracted, which gives the amount of blood by the following formula: 1 mL = 1gm.

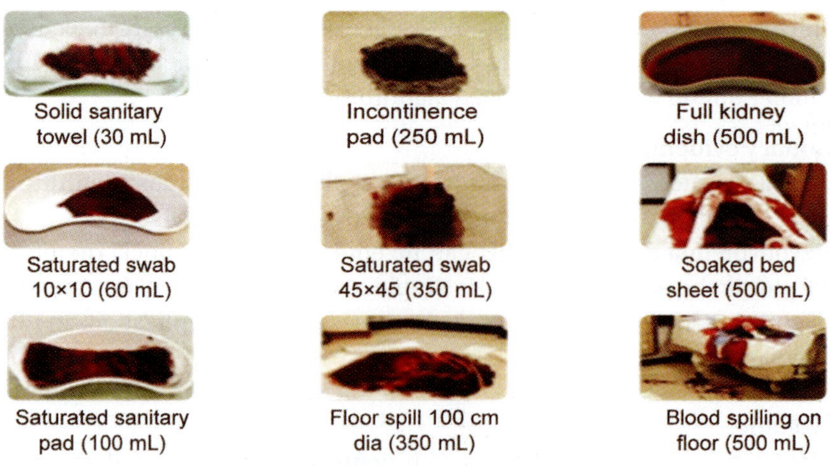

Fig. 1: Visual blood loss volume estimation.

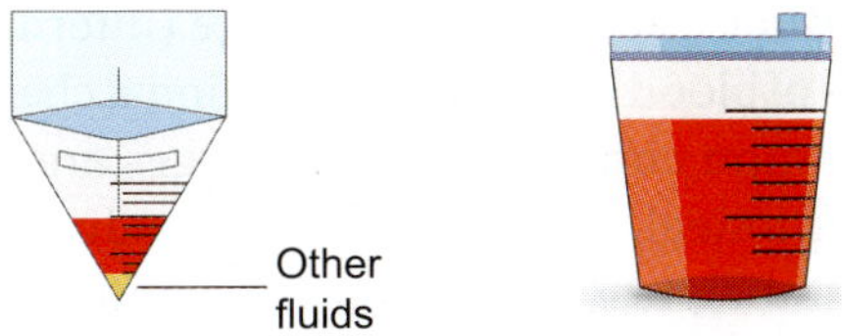

Fig. 2: Calibrated under buttock bags and suction jar for QBL.

Some tips for QBL (use a digital weighing scale):

Subtractors:

- Check the volume before the delivery of placenta in the suction/under-buttock bags
- Any liquid used for cleaning and the amniotic fluid volume

Additions:

- All soaked mops/cloths/sponges/sheets weight change should be added.
- Mops damps with normal saline contain minimal fluid and saline used is already in suction bottle.

Example: 750 mL fluid available in the under-buttock pouch and 200 mL was there before the delivery of placenta and Mops weight difference is 90 g then blood loss calculation will the 750 – 200 + 90 = 640 mL.

Q4. How do we stage or define severity of PPH and what are the various clinical parameters and cut-off values for acute PPH?

Draft recommendations: Obstetric shock indexing and mean arterial pressure are simple, rapid, and better quantitative measure for assessing significant loss and staging the PPH than, quantitative measurement of blood loss in all maternity hospitals as it helps in early diagnosis and timely interventions or referrals in resource limited settings. Obstetricians must have high index of suspicion of hemodynamic susceptibility based on OSI in immediate postpartum period and should be prioritized for close monitoring and it can predict adverse outcomes of PPH.

Evidence summary: An abnormal OSI is an early marker of hemodynamic instability because PPH causes an early elevation of the heart rate driven by baroreceptor reflex-mediated sympathetic activation, aimed at maintaining normal blood pressure, well-before the blood pressure begins to fall. Association of Women's Health, Obstetric and Neonatal Nurses (AWHONN) and California Maternal Quality Care Collaborative (CMQCC) (2015) recommend MEOWS for early identification of PPH and its severity and to reduce inaccuracies that can cause potential delays in decision-making and response to postpartum hemorrhage.

Drawbacks with QBL: Concealed hemorrhage (internal bleeding without outward appearance of blood loss) creates additional challenges for diagnosis and treatment. Common concealed hemorrhages are intra-uterine, intra-abdominal, retroperitoneal, broad ligament bleeding or hematomas and often are difficult to diagnose clinically. The clinical vital monitoring, or scoring method like MEOWS are the savior in absence of visible blood loss **(Table 3)**.

- *Clinical parameters* and their cut-off values of hypovolemia (indirect grading of PPH):
- *Blood pressure (BP):* Systolic <90 mm Hg, or reduction in systolic BP by >40 mm Hg

Mean arterial pressure <70 mm Hg or requirement of inotropic support indicates hypovolemia.

Mean arterial pressure (MAP) = DP + 1/3 (SP – DP) or MAP = DP + 1/3 (PP). Mean arterial pressure (MAP) is a widely accepted target as a clinical determinant of organ perfusion and minimum target MAP of at least 65 mm Hg be maintained by fluid and blood infusion.

Obstetric shock index (OSI) = It is the ratio of heart rate to systolic blood pressure and has a normal range of 0.7–0.9, and higher values without apparent blood loss is suggestive of occult shock. It is the best guide for

TABLE 3: AWHONN-PPH risk prediction model.

Physiological parameter	3	2	1	0	1	2	3
Respiratory rate	<12			12–20		21–25	>25
Oxygen saturations	<92	92–95		>95			
Any supplemental oxygen		Yes		No			
Temperature	<36			36.1–37.2		37.3–37.7	>37.7
Systolic BP	<90			90–140	141–150	151–160	>160
Diastolic BP				60–90	91–100	101–110	>110
Heart rate	<50	50–60		61–100	101–110	111–120	>120
Level of consciousness				A			V, P, or U
Pain (excluding labor)				Normal			Abnormal
Discharge/lochia				Normal			Abnormal
Proteinuria						+	++>

(AWHONN-PPH: Association of Women's Health, Obstetric and Neonatal Nurses; PPH: postpartum hemorrhage)

transfusion requirement. OSI is good for low-resource settings where point-of-care testing (POCT) technology as ABG, base deficit is not available.

Study suggests that women having antepartum hemorrhage (aPR 2.63, $p=0.010$) and having a blood loss just greater than 200 mL (aPR 1.59, $p=0.018$) were significantly associated with abnormal OSI (>0.9), while most definitions take the cut-off of 500 mL for PPH in vaginal delivery.

MEOWS guides safe escalation and de-escalation be used in routinely in maternity centers for early diagnosis, intervention/referral. It is simple, color coded, quantifiable, and has alert (yellow) zones.

Artificial intelligence (AI): This platforms appear promising recently for quantifying blood loss by using mobile technology and image recognition algorithms.

Rule of 30 states that if there is fall in SBP by 30 mm Hg, if the pulse rate increases by at least 30 bpm, if the respiratory rate increases to >30 breaths/min, if the urine output reduces to <30 mL/h, if the hematocrit is <30%, then the amount of blood loss is >30% of the blood volume (approximate 1,500 mL and beyond).

Q5. Other terminologies related to PPH and relation to comorbidities as anemia, preeclampsia, and various anesthetic agents and methods. Do definitions and terminologies in PPH require any considerations in relation delivery mode and comorbidities?

Draft recommendations: Blood loss should not be defined by type (vaginal, forceps, ventouse, cephalic, breech) or mode of delivery (abdominal/vaginal) but by the quantification or clinical vital compromise (covers any concealed hemorrhage too).

- Standardized terminology should be used in documentation.
- Certain comorbidities increase the chances of PPH but standardized definitions and PPH severity should not be changed due to them.

Other terminologies:

Atonic PPH: Term is not clearly defined but refers to prolonged or persistent bleeding that lasts beyond the typical timeframe of acute PPH. Blood loss is not that speedy but continues at a continuous or intermittent phase even beyond 7 days of delivery.

Refractory PPH: Refers to severe bleeding that persists or recurs despite initial treatment and management efforts, requires aggressive and multimodal management in combination.

- Administration of uterotonic agents (e.g., oxytocin, carbetocin, methergine, misoprostol)
- Fluid resuscitation and blood transfusion
- Surgical interventions (e.g., uterine artery ligation, hysterectomy)

Recurrent PPH: Bleeding after the initial control, typically within the first few hours to days after delivery. Retained fragments, pseudoaneurysm, and infection are the common reasons.

Concealed/occult PPH: Bleeding is not appreciated externally but occurs internally. It has maximal diagnostic dilemma and delay. The common causes causing the delay in the diagnosis is due to the false perceptions in the mind of health care team and the known and undetected comorbidities in the patient. Quantification is not at all possible and clinical vital parameters are the only savior. Any MEOWS change not responding to the initial fluid resuscitation should make maternity team alert for the possibility of concealed hemorrhage and Point of Care Ultrasound (POCUS) bed side sonography be planned.

Concealed hemorrhage is caused by loosened vascular ligature, unrecognized laceration of vessels, setting of coagulopathy, extension of cervical laceration, vaginal hematoma, vulval hematoma, or episiotomy hematoma. Delay in the diagnosis occurs by thought that pain is common on first postoperative/delivery day (of uterine contraction), fall in BP (due to regional anesthesia—spinal), confounders like anemia, cardiac disease preeclampsia have tachycardia, etc. Operative field appears dry as intraoperative blood pressure is kept low and present with abdominal bleed in postoperative ward.

PPH and comorbidities:

Anesthesia and PPH: General anesthesia during the C-section or manual removal of placenta makes woman prone for PPH as well as hypotension due to smooth muscle relaxant use leading into uterine atony. Regional anesthesia like spinal, epidural are better in respect that patient remains conscious and PPH risk is less but hypotension is common and high spinal can lead to respiratory compromise too. Combined spinal-epidural have more benefits while limiting the complications.

Anemia and PPH:

- Anemia leads to sympathetic activation and thus causing tachycardia and increased stroke volume further increasing blood loss
- Reduced blood flow from anemia increases the blood flow in the vessels
- Clots formed in anemic patients are more susceptible to hemolysis.
- Anemia causes poor oxygenation of the uterine muscle leading to atony

Preeclampsia and PPH: Preeclampsia has intravascular volume compromise and leaking capillaries in all body systems thus minimal PPH ends up in sudden shock. Load on heart is already increased in PE due to raise BP, systemic vascular resistance, vasospasm, and generalized edema which hampers the contractility of myometrium and exaggerates the chances of PPH multiple fold. Managing PPH in a preeclamptic or eclamptic case is further challenging due to fluid disbalances, coagulopathy, raised blood pressure and leaky capillaries therefore alert mode should be kept for 48 hours postdelivery.

Obesity and PPH: Morbid obesity (BMI > 40%) is an independent risk factor for PPH. Obesity contributes by uterine atony and other challenges as difficult procedural manipulations and position changes, surgical intervention and in sonographic evaluation due to large panniculus.

Q6. Can there be any predictive risk scoring for high-risk identification of PPH prior to delivery workable at low-resource settings so that better planning be proposed?

Draft recommendations: Maternity health centers should use risk scoring model for prediction of PPH at the time of admission in labor and immediately post-partum as it makes provider remain prepared or timely referred from low-resource settings.

Evidence summary: There is always a relationship between hemorrhage risk score and hemorrhage associated morbidity. The AWHONN–PPH risk assessment tool has emerged as a simple, easy to implement, and low-cost hemorrhage-risk prediction tool as women in high risk category were six times more likely to have PPH compared to low risk **(Table 4)**.

If two or more medium risk items are found, then that classifies as "high risk".

TABLE 4: AWOHNN – Association of Women's Health, Obstetric and Neonatal Nurses.

Low risk	*Medium risk*	*High risk*
• No previous uterine incision • Singleton pregnancy • No medical disorder • No known bleeding disorder • No history of PPH • Optimal hemoglobin	• Induction of labor (with oxytocin) or cervical ripening • Multiple gestations • >4 previous vaginal birth • Prior cesarean birth or prior uterine incision • Large uterine fibroids • History of one previous PPH • Family history in first-degree relatives who experienced PPH (known or unknown etiology with possible coagulopathy) • Chorioamnionitis • Fetal demise • Polyhydramnios • Age >35 years • Post ART pregnancy • Dysfunctional labor	• Has two or more medium-risk actors • Active bleeding is more than a "bloody show" • Suspected placenta accrete or percreta • Placenta previa, low-lying placenta • Known coagulopathy • History of more than one previous PPH • Hematocrit <30 and other risk factors • Platelets <100,000/mm^3 • Obstructed labor • Retained placenta • INR >1.5

PPH risk assessment tools have been defined based on pre-pregnancy condition. Routine variables like parity, fetal macrosomia, mode of delivery and history of PPH can predict PPH and nomogram could help in clinical decision-making.

BIBLIOGRAPHY

1. Agaba DC, Lugobe HM, Migisha R, et al. Abnormal obstetric shock index and associated factors among immediate postpartum women following vaginal delivery at a tertiary hospital in southwestern Uganda. BMC Pregnancy Childbirth. 2024;24:31.
2. Al Kadri HM, Al Anazi BK, Tamim HM. Visual estimation versus gravimetric measurement of postpartum blood loss: a prospective cohort study. Arch Gynecol Obstet. 2011;283:1207-13.
3. AWHONN. Quantification of blood loss: AWHONN practice brief number 1. J Obstet Gynecol Neonatal Nurs. 2015;44(1):158-60.
4. Bell SF, Watkins A, John M, et al. Incidence of postpartum haemorrhage defined by quantitative blood loss measurement: a national cohort. BMC Pregnancy Childbirth. 2020;20(1):271.
5. Boujarzadeh B, Ranjbar A, Banihashaemi F, et al. Machine learning approach to predict postpartum haemorrhage: a systematic review protocol. BMJ Open. 2023;13:e067661.
6. Colalillo EL, Sparks AD, Phillips JM, et al. Obstetric haemorrhage risk assessment tool predicts composite maternal morbidity, Sci Rep. 2021;11(1):14709.
7. Diaz V, Abalos E, Carroli, G. Methods for blood loss estimation after vaginal birth. Cochrane Database Syst Rev. 2018;(9):CD010980.
8. FIGO. (2022). Postpartum Haemorrhage Clinical Protocol and Care Pathways. [online] Available from https://www.figo.org/sites/default/files/2022-04/FIGO%20generic%20protocols%20PPH%20%20April%202022.pdf. [Last accessed November, 2024]
9. Menard MK, Main EK, Currigan SM. Executive summary of the reVITALize initiative: standardizing obstetric data definitions. Obstet Gynecol. 2014;124:150-3.
10. Mutschler M, Nienaber U, Brockamp T, et al. A critical reappraisal of the ATLS classification of hypovolaemic shock: Does it really reflect clinical reality? Resuscitation. 2013;84(3):309-13.
11. Mutschler M, Nienaber U, Münzberg M, et al. The Shock Index revisited – a fast guide to transfusion requirement? A retrospective analysis on 21,853 patients derived from the TraumaRegister DGU®. Crit Care. 2013;17:R172.
12. Nathan HL, Seed PT, Hezelgrave NL, et al. Shock index thresholds to predict adverse outcomes in maternal haemorrhage and sepsis: a prospective cohort study. Acta Obstet Gynecol Scand. 2019;98(9):1178-86.
13. Po LK, Simons ME, Levinsky ES. Concealed postpartum haemorrhage treated with transcatheter arterial embolization. Obstet Gynecol. 2012;120(2 Pt 2):461-4.

14. Rath WH. Postpartum haemorrhage—update on problems of definitions and diagnosis. Acta Obstet Gynecol Scand. 201;90(5):421-8.
15. WHO. (2023). WHO announces the first meeting of the postpartum haemorrhage (PPH) bundle Guideline Development Subgroup. [online] Available from https:// www.who.int/news/item/14-08-2023-who-announces-the-first-meeting-of-the-postpartum-haemorrhage-(pph)-bundle-guideline-development-subgroup. [Last accessed November, 2024]

4

CHAPTER

Risk Identification of Postpartum Hemorrhage

Haresh Doshi, Shalini Gainder

Q1. What are the risk factors for PPH?

Draft recommendations: The risk factors should be determined antenatally or as and when arise and patient place of delivery determined accordingly or she may be transported to a place where PPH protocol can be followed **(Table 1)**.

Woman undergoing cesarean section for any of the above-mentioned risk factors identified antenatally or with failed progress of labor are considered at risk of PPH. In cesarean births, delivery after full dilation is a risk factor

TABLE 1: Risk factors for postpartum hemorrhage.

Antenatal	***In labor***	***During cesarean***	***Postpartum***
Previous PPH	Induction of labor	Previous uterine incision	Chorioamnionitis
Previous retained placenta	Prolonged Ist, IInd or IIIrd stage of labor	Known bleeding disorder	Platelets <1 lakh/mm^3 INR >1.5
Maternal anemia	Secondary arrest of labor	Large uterine fibroids	Known coagulopathy
Maternal age (>35 years or more)	Use of oxytocin	IInd stage cesarean	Obstructed labor
Body mass index greater than 35 kg/m^2	Precipitate labor	Placenta accreta or percreta	Retained products
Grand multiparity	Operative delivery	Placenta previa	
Antepartum hemorrhage	Cesarean section	Known coagulopathy	
Over distention of the uterus	Chorioamnionitis	Chorioamnionitis	
Pre-existing uterine abnormalities	Known bleeding disorder	Obstructed labor	
	Large uterine fibroids	Post ART Pregnancy	
	Platelets <1 lakh/mm^3 INR >1.5		

for unintended uterine incision extension, particularly in the setting of past cesarean birth or failed instrumental delivery attempt.

Summary of evidence: In a systematic review by Ende HB et al. included a number of population-based studies are available from different population groups and different geographical areas. It says that most cases of PPH have no identifiable risk factors. Multivariate logistic regression models were developed to examine the maternal characteristic associated with severe PPH, features and complications of the pregnancy and birth, and the management of labor. The data was analyzed and the risk assessment and odd's ratio calculated for each risk factors and based on these studies as evidence the risk factors were included above.

Q2. Are risk factors increasing in modern times?

Draft recommendations: There is increase in the PPH in present era attributable to rises in the incidence of several key risk factors, including previous cesarean section, labor induction and augmentation, placenta previa, and abnormal placentation. The recent increase in maternal age of primigravida's and use of IVF technology has a paradigm shift to pregnancies in third and fourth decade of life which are more complicated with PPH. The PAS is newer aspect of critical care in obstetrics and incidence is increasing due to more cases of cesarean sections.

Summary of evidence: Literature review was done to assess the changing trends in the women who had PPH and emerging new trends were reported in recent studies

Research gap: Most of the evidence is based on the retrospective cohort studies and no randomized control studies are available to strengthen the evidence.

Q3. Are risk factors same for all the ethnic groups?

Draft recommendations: The risk for PPH can vary among different population groups either based on ethnicity which impacts the body habitus due to obesity. Ethnic variation can impact their instinct to seek antenatal care or place of delivery which can also be impacted by their socioeconomic, demographic, and education level.

Ethnic minorities and Hispanic population are prone to atonic PPH compared to Caucasians. The genetic risk factors to develop gestational diabetes and hypertension can impact the ethnic variability to develop PPH. The presence of hemoglobinopathies in certain ethnic minorities can increase the incidence of PPH. Sometimes different risks in different ethnic groups may be due to variation in labor practices and cultural differences.

Summary of evidence: Risk factors for different ethnic groups are reported in some recent studies. Okunlola O et al. said genetic susceptibility to both atony and other risk factors like hypertension or diabetes in specific patient populations may also explain this association.

Q4. How much risk assessment tool is useful for prediction of PPH?

Draft recommendations: Most women who develop PPH have no predictive factor and despite the low predictive value of current risk assessment tools, use of a tool is better than no risk assessment as the risk stratification process may raise consciousness and preparation.

Summary of evidence: The California Maternal Quality Care Collaborative (CMQCC) involving Lagrew D et al. recommends intrapartum obstetric hemorrhage risk assessment on admission to the labor unit, at the start of the second stage of labor, at transfer to postpartum care, and any time the patient's condition changes.

A systematic review of 14 prognostic models for PPH by Neary C et al. reported that none were adequately validated in the general obstetric population, three were useful in patients undergoing cesarean birth, patients with placenta previa or placenta accreta spectrum. A study compared the predictive value of the CMQCC, American College of Obstetricians and Gynecologists Safe Motherhood Initiative (ACOG SMI), and Association of Women's Health, Obstetric and Neonatal Nurses (AWOHNN), PPH risk stratification tools in over 11,000 patients concluded that none performed sufficiently well for predicting PPH.

CMQCC toolkit: The CMQCC risk classification scheme is used initially for patients admitted to the labor unit. It classifies patients as low, medium, or high risk for PPH, in a validation study of an earlier version (version 1.0 in 2010), the incidence of severe PPH (i.e., necessitating transfusion) in the three groups was 0.8, 2.0, and 7.3 percent, respectively, and only 22 percent of severe PPH cases occurred in high-risk group. The CMQCC tool provides for ongoing risk assessment by including intrapartum and postpartum risk factors in the checklist.

BIBLIOGRAPHY

1. Ende HB, Lozada MJ, Chestnut DH, et al. Risk factors for atonic postpartum hemorrhage: a systematic review and meta-analysis. Obstet Gynecol. 2021; 137(2):305-23.
2. Lagrew D, McNulty J, Sakowski C, et al. (2022). Improving health care response to obstetric hemorrhage: a California Maternal Quality Care Collaborative toolkit. [online] Available from https://www.cmqcc.org/sites/default/files/HEMToolkit_03252022%20Errata%207.2022%20%282%29.pdf. [Last accessed November, 2024]

3. Neary C, Naheed S, McLernon DJ, et al. Predicting risk of postpartum haemorrhage: a systematic review. BJOG. 2021;128(1):46-53.
4. Okunlola O, Raza S, Osasan S. Race/ethnicity as a risk factor in the development of postpartum hemorrhage: a thorough systematic review of disparity in the relationship between pregnancy and the rate of postpartum hemorrhage. Cureus. 2022;14(6):e26460.

CHAPTER 5

Prevention of Postpartum Hemorrhage

Madhva Prasad, Sushil Chawla

"Learn cutting-edge prevention techniques that save lives."

- **Briefing:**
  - Antenatal care recommendations to reduce risk
  - Medications and interventions during labor to prevent PPH
- **Unanswered Questions:**
  - What are the potential roles of emerging technologies such as wearable devices in the prevention of PPH?
  - How can community-based interventions be better designed to address the prevention of PPH in remote areas?
- **Recommendations**

Q1. What are the interventions in antenatal period for prevention of PPH?

Draft recommendations: Early introduction and regular antenatal care services play a critical role in reducing postpartum hemorrhage. Prevention, early identification, and prompt management of antenatal risk factors like a range of conditions like prepartum anemia, hypertension and related complications, placenta previa, adherent placenta, macrosomia, diabetes and intrauterine fetal death, etc. play an indirect role in reducing postpartum hemorrhage.

Evidence summary: Large comparative studies have highlighted the associations between lack of adequate antenatal care and occurrence of postpartum hemorrhage. Due to inadequate antenatal care, conditions like prepartum anemia, hypertension and related complications, placenta previa, adherent placenta, macrosomia, intrauterine fetal demise (eventual) may be missed. When these conditions are not adequately tackled in the antenatal period, they appear to have an indirect compound effect and lead to higher occurrence of postpartum hemorrhage.

Q2A. What are the interventions in the 1st stage of labor for prevention of PPH?

Draft recommendations: Clinicians must be aware that induction of labor, immaterial of method, may be associated with increase in PPH. Induction of labor should be chosen judiciously and carefully.

Evidence summary: Induction of labor is a commonly performed intervention. While analyzing risk benefits, the higher risk of PPH must be taken into account (an odds ratio of 1.56 for PPH and odds ratio of 1.51 for severe PPH). While it may be acknowledged that the reason for induction of labor may be an obstetric condition, which may also contribute to the development of PPH, some analytical results suggest the persistence of association even after adjusting for these confounding factors. Whereas, some have noted that elective induction at 39 weeks does not give rise to any increase in PPH.

Draft recommendations: Clinicians must be aware that usage of oxytocin for labor augmentation is associated with a slight increase in PPH. Judicious and careful usage of oxytocin in monitored and supervised environments is crucial for prevention of PPH.

Evidence summary: Initially, it was believed that usage of oxytocin does not increase PPH risk as long as AMTSL is performed. Later, questions were raised about the validity of the evidence regarding utility of various uterotonic agents for prevention of PPH among deliveries which occurred after oxytocin augmentation. Hence, the data from major trials on PPH were reanalyzed. Such analysis has suggested a strong association between oxytocin augmentation and occurrence of PPH. An incremental association between dosage and duration of oxytocin usage and occurrence of PPH has also been noted. Clinicians and institutions must draw tailored protocols balancing urgency of delivery and risk of PPH. Whether a balanced and calculated avoidance of oxytocin augmentation can reduce the occurrence of PPH is an unanswered question.

Draft recommendations: If labor was induced or augmented, and active stage of 1st stage of labor has been definitely reached, discontinuation of augmenting agent can be considered.

Evidence summary: A 2022 updated systematic review meta-analysis gives a risk ratio of 0.78 for the occurrence of PPH among those whose oxytocin was discontinued after the attainment of active stage of 1st stage of labor. Among other benefits (like lesser conversion of cesarean section etc.), a slight reduction of postpartum hemorrhage has been noted.

Q2B. What are the interventions in 2nd stage of labor for prevention of PPH?

Draft recommendations: Clinicians must be aware that women with weak uterine contractions, a prolonged second stage of labor (more than 2 hours), and a more prolonged pushing time are at higher propensity for PPH.

Evidence summary: An updated meta-analysis shows women with weaker uterine contractions having higher risk of PPH compared to those with normal contractions (27.5% vs. 18.5%, relative risk of 1.6, *p* value <0.01). Those with second stage labor duration more than 2 hours had higher risk of PPH (34.5% vs. 15.9%, relative risk of 0.20, *p* value <0.01). Whether interventions to reduce second stage of labor will result in reduction of PPH remains largely unanswered. A large cohort study showed that there was an association between duration of pushing and occurrence of PPH. While instrumental delivery can per se increase the risk of PPH, such instrumentation performed after 3 hours of 2nd stage of labor has much higher risk of PPH.

Draft recommendations: There is no clarity regarding continuation or discontinuation of oxytocin in the 2nd stage of labor.

Evidence summary: A large retrospective cohort analyzed that PPH occurred in 15.2% of those who stopped oxytocin and 5.7% who continued oxytocin. However, this analysis was immaterial of mode of delivery. Among those who went for LSCS, PPH rates were 38% and 36%, whereas among those who went for cesarean delivery, PPH rates were lesser in the stopped oxytocin group (3.8% vs. 5.2%). Since it is difficult to predict which patient may end up needing cesarean section, there is, at present, no clarity regarding whether to continue or discontinue oxytocin in 2nd stage of labor, from prevention of PPH point of view.

Q2C. What are the interventions in the 3rd stage of labor for prevention of PPH?

The following recommendations are drafted using the latest guidelines advocated by FIGO, WHO and FOGSI, as appropriate.

Draft recommendations:

- Active management of the third stage of labor (AMTSL) reduces the occurrence of severe postpartum hemorrhage by approximately 60–70%.
- The use of uterotonics for prevention of PPH during the third stage of labor is recommended for all births, both vaginal and cesarean delivery.
- Combination therapies are acceptable methods for prevention of PPH
- Oxytocin [10 IU intravenously/intramuscularly (IV/IM)] is recommended within one minute of the delivery of the baby after excluding the second twin.
- In settings where oxytocin is used, attention should be paid to the oxytocin cold chain (2 to 8 degrees).
- Carbetocin (heat stable) 100 microgram IM/IV is recommended for the prevention of PPH.
- If oxytocin and methylergometrine combination is chosen, intramuscular methylergometrine (0.2 mg) and intravenous oxytocin (10 IU) immediately after delivery of the neonate are recommended.

- If oxytocin is unavailable or its quality cannot be guaranteed, the use of other injectable uterotonics (if appropriate ergometrine/methylergometrine 200 μg IM/IV; hypertensive disorders, cardiac disease, and severe anemia can be safely excluded prior to its use) or oral misoprostol (400–600 μg orally) or carbetocin 100 μg IM/IV is recommended for the prevention of PPH.
- If oxytocin and tranexamic acid combination is chosen, intravenous tranexamic acid (1 g) in addition to intravenous oxytocin (10 IU) immediately after delivery of the neonate and before placental delivery is recommended.
- If oxytocin and misoprostol combination is chosen, sublingual misoprostol (400 μg) in addition to intravenous oxytocin (10 IU) immediately after delivery of the neonate is recommended.
- Controlled cord traction after seeing signs of placental separation by skilled birth attendant to avoid inversion
- Avoid inserting hand inside the uterus as it leads to endomyometritis.
- Sustained uterine massage is not recommended as an intervention to prevent PPH in women who have received prophylactic oxytocin.
- Postpartum abdominal uterine tone assessment for early identification of uterine atony is recommended for all women.
- Delayed cord clamping (performed after 1 to 3 minutes after birth) is still recommended for all births to reduce newborn anemia while beginning essential newborn care at the same time(unless contraindicated)
- The placenta should be examined for complete removal after delivery.
- There is insufficient evidence to support or refute umbilical cord milking, uterine massage, or nipple stimulation for the prevention of postpartum hemorrhage.

Q3. What are the potential roles of emerging technologies such as wearable devices in the prevention of PPH?

The most common uses for wearable technology (as we stated earlier) are for helping to monitor and alert the wearer about their personal health information or for social communication purposes—like calling, texting, social media, etc. Latest gadgets like watches and bands can detect hypotension, tachycardia, ECG, SpO_2, and alert the health care team during monitoring and transfer of the patient to the higher center.

Q4. How can community-based interventions be better designed to address the prevention of PPH in remote areas?

Draft recommendations: In remote areas, community settings, noninstitutional settings, where birth attendants with skills of administering intramuscular injections are available, provision of basic medications like oxytocin should be ensured by identifying resources earmarked for storage of oxytocin and maintaining cold chain. Where cold chain compromise is a possibility, heat stable oxytocin should be considered. Where birth attendants do not have injection skills, usage of oral misoprostol can be enhanced by advance distribution of misoprostol during the late trimester antenatal visits, with due education.

Evidence summary: Availability of uterotonic drugs is a major limiting factor in the effective prevention and treatment of postpartum hemorrhage. Adequate evidence is available regarding the positive benefits of making appropriate drugs locally available, and even providing oral medications in the hands of the end user. Various factors identified as problems in effective implementation of this strategy were inconsistency in supplies and its distribution; inadequate staffing; lack of knowledge of providers and end users, absence of the registration of drug and fear and apprehensions related to its use at provider and policy level. The effectiveness has been proven in Indian settings and should be considered where feasible.

Draft recommendations: Best utilization of skilled and unskilled manpower should be considered for the optimal prevention of PPH. Healthcare providers must be aware of concepts like "task-shifting".

Evidence summary: A recent review suggests that even less-well trained attendants can be utilized for activities like uterine massage, measurement of vital parameters, etc., while slightly more technical activities like controlled cord traction should be done by trained clinicians. The stratification of activities and effective utilization of manpower is a key concept in prevention of PPH.

Draft recommendations: The implementation of programs for prevention of obstetric hemorrhage at the community level should focus on prophylactic use of uterotonics, enhancement of clinical provider skills training, provision of clinical guidelines and multi-component quality improvement bundles.

Evidence summary: Ensuring the availability of optimal prenatal care, detection of high risk cases, intrapartum care is necessary to reduce the aftermaths of this condition on the society.

There has been poor penetration of community efforts for prevention of PPH. How to better improve the penetration and sustainability of already drafted guidelines in the community setting, so as to effectively reach the end-user is a question that needs to be answered more clearly.

BIBLIOGRAPHY

1. ACOG Committee Opinion. Quantitative blood loss in obstetric hemorrhage: ACOG Committee Opinion, Number 794. Obstet Gynecol. 2019;134(6):e150-6.
2. Akter S, Forbes G, Vazquez Corona M, et al. Perceptions and experiences of the prevention, detection, and management of postpartum haemorrhage:

a qualitative evidence synthesis. Cochrane Database Syst Rev. 2023;11(11): CD013795.

3. Althabe F, Therrien MNS, Pingray V, et al. Postpartum hemorrhage care bundles to improve adherence to guidelines: a WHO technical consultation. Int J Gynecol Obstet. 2020;148:290-9.
4. American College of Obstetricians and Gynecologists. Clinical management guidelines for obstetrician-gynecologists: postpartum hemorrhage. ACOG Practice Bulletin No. 183. Obstet Gynecol. 2017;130(4):e168-86.
5. Association of Women's Health, Obstetric and Neonatal Nurses (AWHONN). Obstetric patient safety: Consensus bundle on postpartum hemorrhage. J Obstet Gynecol Neonat Nurs. 2014;43(4):462-5.
6. Brenner A, Shakur-Still H, Chaudhri R, et al. The impact of early outcome events on the effect of tranexamic acid in post-partum haemorrhage: an exploratory subgroup analysis of the WOMAN trial. BMC Pregnancy Childbirth. 2018; 18:215.
7. Escobar M, Nassar AH, Theron G, et al. FIGO recommendations on the management of postpartum hemorrhage 2022. Int J Gynaecol Obstet. 2022;157 (Suppl 1): 3-50.
8. Kumari SS. (2022). FOGSI: PPH prevention and management. Updated PPH guidelines. September 2022. [online] Available from https://www.fogsi. org/ wp-content/uploads/tog/pph-prevention-and-management-updated-sept-2022.pdf. [Last accessed November, 2024]
9. Mavrides E, Allard S, Chandraharan E, et al. Prevention and management of postpartum haemorrhage. BJOG. 2016;124:e106-1498.
10. Parry Smith WR, Papadopoulou A, Thomas E, et al. Uterotonic agents for first-line treatment of postpartum haemorrhage: a network meta-analysis. Cochrane Database Syst Rev. 2020;(11):CD012754.
11. Perel P, Roberts I, Ker K. Colloids versus crystalloids for fluid resuscitation in critically ill patients. Cochrane Database Syst Rev. 2013;(2):CD000567.
12. Robinson D, Basso M, Chan C, et al. Guideline No. 431: Postpartum hemorrhage and hemorrhagic shock. J Obstet Gynaecol Can. 2022;44(12):1293-310.e1.
13. Royal College of Midwives. Evidence-based guidelines for midwifery-led care in labour: postpartum haemorrhage. Brit J Midwifery. 2012;20(5):321-8.
14. Ryan N, Vieira D, Goffman D, et al. Implementation outcomes of policy and programme innovations to prevent obstetric haemorrhage in low- and middle-income countries: a systematic review. Health Policy Plan. 2020;35(9):1208-27.
15. WHO. WHO recommendations for the prevention and treatment of postpartum haemorrhage. Geneva: World Health Organization; 2012.

6

CHAPTER

Medical Management of Postpartum Hemorrhage

Latha Venkataram, Srimathy Raman, Mrutyunjaya Bellad, Vidyadhar Bangal

"Optimize patient outcomes with streamlined medical protocols."

Q1. Who are the personnel needed in the management of PPH and their individual roles and responsibilities?

Draft recommendations: Effective management of postpartum hemorrhage (PPH)—especially major PPH requires a coordinated multidisciplinary team approach. Each member of the team has specific roles and responsibilities to ensure timely and efficient management of PPH.

Evidence: It is important that there is an early involvement of appropriate senior staff in management of PPH, especially major PPH. The multidisciplinary team (MDT) team includes obstetrician/s, nurses/midwives, anesthesiologists, intensivists, blood bank and hematologist (MTP), and support staff. Each member should have a specific task and role assigned to them. The obstetrician leads the management team. He/she is generally tasked with the management of the cause of hemorrhage and is responsible for performing appropriate steps including escalation of care and surgical interventions, if necessary (e.g., uterine balloon tamponade, suturing, or hysterectomy).

The nurses/midwives are usually the first responders and perform the initial assessment and management and lend able support to the obstetrician in performing measures like uterine massage, monitoring, administration of uterotonics, organizing investigations, blood and blood products.

The anesthesiologist/intensivist plays an important role in the assessment and management of airway, breathing, and circulation—hemodynamic stabilization and provides anesthesia for surgical interventions.

The blood bank personnel and the hematologist play an important role in the massive transfusion situations, provide inputs, and ensure timely provision of blood and components.

The support staff play a critical role in documentation and assisting with patient care and patient transport to operating room or intensive care unit. In case of need for transfer to higher center, equipped ambulance with required personnel and co-ordination with the MDT in the higher center is important.

The collaboration and coordination among these team members are essential for the effective management of PPH and ensuring the best possible outcomes for the patient.

Q2. What are principles of management of PPH?

Draft recommendations: Remember the Golden hour—quick and efficient management is extremely important to avoid mortality and morbidity. The goals are to resuscitate, implement specific measures for the cause and communicate effectively.

ABCDE approach should be followed for resuscitation with an appropriate and early involvement of multidisciplinary team.

Hemostatic resuscitation with careful balance of crystalloids, colloids, blood, and blood products is important.

Evaluation of the hemodynamic status and etiology of PPH should happen simultaneously with institution of resuscitation measures and management of the cause.

Evidence: Evidence has shown that 88% of deaths occur in the first 2–4 hours of PPH. WOMAN trial showed that even at the time of PPH diagnosis, 60% of patients had clinical signs of hemodynamic instability and 4% had signs of end-organ damage. This points out to the importance of early diagnosis and intervention in the golden hour.

The management principles are resuscitation/control of bleeding/restoration of circulating blood volume—remembered by the mnemonic ORDER: Oxygenate, Restore circulating volume, drug therapy, Evaluate response to therapy, Remedy underlying cause. It is important to avoid the "lethal triad" of coagulopathy, acidosis, and hypothermia.

PPH is an obstetric emergency and all PPH guidelines place emphasis on a multidisciplinary team approach. The first step is to call for help and act in a coordinated manner with MDT.

All PPH guidelines advise on ABCDE approach for resuscitation and stabilization and treatment specific to the cause of PPH.

- Airway maintenance (if impaired consciousness due to shock); avoid hypothermia
- Supplementation of oxygen at a flow rate of 10–15 L/min via a facemask (irrespective of maternal oxygenation)
- Intravenous access/vital signs/investigations/volume infusion

Placement and maintenance of two large IV cannula (preferably 16/18 gauge); blood investigations (full blood count, coagulation screen, urea and electrolytes, blood grouping and cross-matching; consider ABG, electrolytes, LFT).

Point-of-care tests—viscoelastic hemostatic assays (VHA)—TEG and ROTEM are now used in PPH to detect coagulation abnormalities as well as to guide blood product replacements. They are used commonly in the management of other intraoperative and trauma-related bleeding as there is evidence showing a decrease in the need for transfusion though major clinical benefits have not been noted. In PPH, there has been no consistent evidence of the benefit of VHA based treatment. This is because of a lack of pregnancy-specific reference values and algorithms apart from the expense.

Monitoring vital parameters like heart rate (HR), blood pressure (BP), respiratory rate, and peripheral oxygen saturation and urine output monitoring is important. MEOWS charting is a useful tool to alert regarding abnormal trends and this has been stressed in multiple confidential enquiries.

Fluid resuscitation is a critical aspect to maintain the circulation. Hence having a large 16/18 Gauge cannula is preferred as the flow rate is 196 with 16 gauge, 90 with 18 gauge, and 61 and 36 respectively with 20- and 22-gauge cannulas.

Fluid resuscitation is initially with crystalloids and colloids. RCOG guideline recommends a maximum of 3.5 L before the start of blood transfusion. This includes up to 2 L crystalloids and if there is delay in availability of blood components the colloids can be considered for the infusion.

Balanced crystalloid solutions such as Ringer's lactate are preferred to saline as there is risk of hyperchloremic acidosis with saline. Evidence is sparse on the ideal fluid as there are no RCTs which have compared the use of colloids with other replacement fluids in PPH. It is important to avoid hypothermia as this exacerbates acidosis and DIC. Hence administration of warmed fluids at 37°C is important.

Administration of crystalloids in boluses of 500 mL is recommended along with dynamic assessment of fluid responsiveness to guide further resuscitation. Measuring IVC diameter could be considered for assessment of hypovolemia and response to fluid replacement invasive measures like arterial line, central venous pressure (CVP), may need to be considered based on individual circumstances.

Early recourse to blood and blood products is important as fluid resuscitation can cause dilutional coagulopathy which will aggravate bleeding. There is no clear evidence on the volume of fluid which would cause this and if this contributes to adverse outcomes. Packed red blood cells are recommended to be administered in a 1:1:1 ratio with fresh frozen plasma (FFP) and platelets.

- Consider drugs—uterotonics/TXA/vasopressors
- Evaluate the cause/response to treatment

It is important to recognize the severity of PPH and recognize the cause at the earliest for efficient management. Careful clinical examination to determine the cause of PPH-4 Ts (Tone, Tissue, Trauma, Thrombin) or combination of Ts should be done simultaneously along with the above measures.

Research gaps: Type of fluids for resuscitation:

- Hypotensive resuscitation
- POC-VHA tests

Q3. What are the different pharmacological measures that can be employed in the management of PPH?

Draft recommendations:

- In atonic PPH, medical methods (single/combination) should be commenced and continued along with mechanical methods.
- Intravenous oxytocin bolus 5 U IV and/or infusion is the first-line uterotonic drug for the treatment of PPH.
- If the bleeding does not respond to oxytocin, second line agents like ergometrine, carboprost, or sublingual misoprostol are recommended.
- Carbetocin is recommended for prevention of PPH.
- Tranexamic acid should be administered early as soon as PPH is diagnosed and is best given within 3 hours of delivery.

Evidence: The initial management of PPH is directed at measures that stimulate myometrial contractions like emptying the bladder, performing uterine massage, bimanual uterine compression, and occasionally even aortic compression while we administer uterotonics.

Uterotonic medications are the first-line medical treatment for atonic PPH. The choice of agent is often based on the side effect profile and provider discretion. Often, we may need to use a combination of multiple agents and a sequence of mechanical and pharmacological measures.

- *Oxytocin:* This is the first-line drug in the medical management of PPH. A repeat bolus of oxytocin 5 IU by slow intravenous injection can be administered. Oxytocin infusion of 40 IU in 500 mL isotonic crystalloids at 125 mL/hour (unless fluid restriction) is then commenced simultaneously. As per FOGSI guidelines, dosage is 20–40 IU in 1 L normal saline, infuse 500 mL over 10 minutes then 250 mL per hour.
- *Carbetocin:* It has not been studied as a therapeutic agent for PPH and so should not be used for treatment. However, if carbetocin is already administered as part of AMTSL, then oxytocin cannot be used as uterotonic for management of PPH. This is due to its equivalent affinity for the oxytocin receptor and long half-life of 40 minutes.
- *Methylergometrine:* 0.2 mg IM/IV every two to four hours (maximum of 5 doses—1 mg) is a potent uterotonic but the side effect profile limits its use as second line. It cannot be used in patients with hypertension, and it can precipitate coronary artery vasospasm and myocardial ischemia.

- *Carboprost:* The recommended dose is 250 micrograms intramuscularly. This may be repeated every 15 minutes to a total dose of 2 mg (eight doses). Its adverse effects like nausea, vomiting, diarrhea, and fever limit its use to a second-line agent. SOGC recommends loperamide to be given concurrently with carboprost to counteract its diarrheal effects. It should not be used in patients with asthma.
- *Misoprostol:* The recommended dose is misoprostol 800 micrograms sublingually. SOGC cautions that it should not be given rectally as the serum levels may not be significant due to poor bioavailability. It is a valuable adjunct to the other agents (oxytocin, ergometrine, carboprost, and TXA) which have a more rapid onset and are useful as independent agents. The side effects are dose dependent, and include shivering, fever, nausea, vomiting, and diarrhea. Further if the above dose of misoprostol has been used for AMTSL or in the management of PPH earlier, there is no evidence on the role of additional misoprostol.
- *Tranexamic acid:* 1 g undiluted IV over 10 minutes (e.g.,1 g/10 mL IV at 1 mL per minute). A repeat dose of a further 1 g can be given after 30 minutes if there is ongoing bleeding. TXA should be administered early in situations where there is a need for a second-line uterotonic. TXA reduced death by 20–30% and was not associated with an increase in adverse effects. It also reduced the need for laparotomy to control bleeding by 36%. It is recommended to be given within 3 hours of delivery and every 15-minute delay resulted in a 10% reduction of TXA efficacy and immediate treatment improved survival by over 70%.

Research gaps: Ideal uterotonic/combination of uterotonics in the management of PPH

Role of carbetocin in treatment of PPH

Q4. How will you modify care in resource-limited settings and care during transfer?

Draft recommendations: The need for transfer to a tertiary care center should be assessed early and resuscitation measures should be continued while transferring.

Measures like balloon tamponade and nonpneumatic antishock garment (NASG) should be considered during transfer.

Evidence: In a resource-limited setting, minimum essential care must be performed as proposed by the PPH first response bundle.

A. Administer oxygen by mask (5–6 L/min) and keep the patient warm
B. Securing IV line and administration of warm intravenous fluid—preferably Ringer's lactate

C. Administration of drugs like repeat oxytocin IV/IM dose, administration of injection tranexamic acid, sublingual administration of tablet misoprostol 800 micrograms.
D. Abdominal uterine massage and ensuring that the uterine cavity is empty and there is no soft tissue injury. Tight vaginal packing should be considered if there is vaginal, cervical, or para-urethral tear and facility for suturing is not available.

Consideration of performing nonsurgical interventions as per PPH refractory bundle like bimanual uterine compression, aortic compression, application of nonpneumatic antishock garment (NASG) and use of uterine balloon tamponade.

WHO and FIGO guidelines recommend use of NASG in PPH especially in women with signs of shock during transport to a tertiary center.

Emergency transport (linked to GPS facility) to the nearest higher center having facility for blood transfusion and surgical intervention should be planned in a well-equipped ambulance (necessary drugs/supplies) with the required medical/paramedical personnel. It is important to ensure that the patient has received adequate resuscitative measures before transfer. Appropriate communication with the staff, patient and the receiving facility and completion of referral slip with all the details (including investigations/treatment) is important.

BIBLIOGRAPHY

1. ACOG Committee Opinion. Quantitative blood loss in obstetric hemorrhage: ACOG Committee Opinion, Number 794. Obstet Gynecol. 2019;134(6):e150-6.
2. Althabe F, Therrien MNS, Pingray V, et al. Postpartum hemorrhage care bundles to improve adherence to guidelines: a WHO technical consultation. Int J Gynecol Obstet. 2020;148:290-9.
3. American College of Obstetricians and Gynecologists. Clinical management guidelines for obstetrician-gynecologists: postpartum hemorrhage. ACOG Practice Bulletin No. 183. Obstet Gynecol. 2017;130(4):e168-86.
4. Association of Women's Health, Obstetric and Neonatal Nurses (AWHONN). Obstetric patient safety: Consensus bundle on postpartum hemorrhage. J Obstet Gynecol Neonat Nurs. 2014;43(4):462-5.
5. Brenner A, Shakur-Still H, Chaudhri R, et al. The impact of early outcome events on the effect of tranexamic acid in post-partum haemorrhage: an exploratory subgroup analysis of the WOMAN trial. BMC Pregnancy Childbirth. 2018; 18:215.
6. Escobar M, Nassar AH, Theron G, et al. FIGO recommendations on the management of postpartum hemorrhage 2022. Int J Gynaecol Obstet. 2022;157 (Suppl 1): 3-50.
7. Kumari SS. (2022). FOGSI: PPH prevention and management. Updated PPH guidelines. September 2022. [online] Available from https://www.fogsi. org/wp-content/uploads/tog/pph-prevention-and-management-updated-sept-2022.pdf. [Last accessed November, 2024]

8. Mavrides E, Allard S, Chandraharan E, et al. Prevention and management of postpartum haemorrhage. BJOG. 2016;124:e106-1498.
9. Parry Smith WR, Papadopoulou A, Thomas E, et al. Uterotonic agents for first-line treatment of postpartum haemorrhage: a network meta-analysis. Cochrane Database Syst Rev. 2020;(11):CD012754.
10. Perel P, Roberts I, Ker K. Colloids versus crystalloids for fluid resuscitation in critically ill patients. Cochrane Database Syst Rev. 2013;(2):CD000567.
11. Robinson D, Basso M, Chan C, et al. Guideline No. 431: Postpartum hemorrhage and hemorrhagic shock. J Obstet Gynaecol Can. 2022;44(12):1293-310.e1.
12. Royal College of Midwives. Evidence-based guidelines for midwifery-led care in labour: postpartum haemorrhage. Brit J Midwifery. 2012;20(5):321-8.
13. WHO. WHO recommendations for the prevention and treatment of postpartum haemorrhage. Geneva: World Health Organization; 2012.

CHAPTER 7

Hemo-resuscitation

BS Susheela Rani

INTRODUCTION

The cornerstone in the management of postpartum hemorrhage (PPH) is managing blood loss. While interventions are being done to identify, assess, and manage the cause for bleeding, appropriate and adequate replacement of blood and its components when required is vital to prevent mortality and morbidity. Timely blood transfusion can save lives; however, inappropriate and improper transfusion can be risky because of complications like hemolytic reactions, TRALI, GVHD, TACO, etc.

Q1. What are the indications for blood transfusion in PPH?

Draft recommendations: Any bleeding obstetric patient with progressively increasing heart rate and falling blood pressures needs blood transfusion.

Summary: In PPH, early decision to replace blood components especially in the setting of ongoing hemorrhage helps to restore hemodynamic balance and minimizes the risk dilutional coagulopathy, electrolyte imbalances, and hypothermia. It is not the amount of blood loss, rather the clinical impact of the blood loss that indicates the need for blood transfusion.

Q2. What is the role of component therapy in PPH?

Draft recommendations:

- There are no uniform guidelines for component therapy in PPH.
- If hemodynamic balance is not restored with transfusion of 2 L of crystalloids, if there is ongoing hemorrhage, 2 units of PRBC is transfused even before the laboratory results on blood parameters are available.
- Subsequent transfusions are based on control of bleeding, clinical evaluation of hemodynamic status, and laboratory results.

Red Blood Cells (RBCs)

Draft recommendations:

- RBCs that are transfused should be ABO and Rh compatible.
- When there is profuse bleeding in PPH, due to urgent requirement, compatibility testing may not be possible.

Types of PRBC available for emergency transfusion:

- When transfusion is required immediately and cannot wait for testing—universal donor (O negative) uncrossmatched RBC

- When transfusion is required before full testing can be completed—group compatible uncrossmatched (type specific) RBC
- Fully crossmatched group and type specific RBC—preferred but takes more than 30 minutes

During transfusion, if the infusion rate is >100 mL/min, a blood warmer is preferable to avoid hypothermia.

Response: After the transfusion of RBCs, the hemoglobin level should equilibrate within 15 minutes of transfusion. One unit should increase the Hb in an average-size patient (70–80 kg) by approximately one g/dL and the hematocrit by 3%.

Fresh Frozen Plasma

Draft recommendations:

Indication: Fresh frozen plasma is used to replace the clotting factors in PPH and to reverse consumptive coagulopathy such as disseminated intravascular coagulation following severe hemorrhage or placental abruption.

If bleeding is continuing and not controlled after transfusion of 2 units of RBC, FFP is administered at a dose of 12–15 mL/kg along with more RBCs to optimize the coagulation factor levels. This dose will raise the level of any factor, including fibrinogen, by close to 30%, which is typically sufficient for hemostasis. Subsequent FFP transfusion should be guided by the results of clotting tests. Once thawed it should be used within 6 hours at room temperature or till 24 hours if kept in refrigerator, at 4°C.

Cryoprecipitate

Draft recommendations: Cryoprecipitate (10–20 mL) contains fibrinogen, Factors VIII, XIII, VWF

Usually available in pools of 5 units and most women need 2 pools (10 units) 2 pools increase fibrinogen by 1 g/dL

FFP and cryoprecipitate should be ABO compatible. Crossmatching tests are usually not performed.

Any D type can be given irrespective of the recipient's D status. Rh D immunoglobulin is not required.

Fibrinogen Concentrate

Draft recommendations:

- Levels of fibrinogen at the time of blood loss are predictive of massive bleeding. A cut-off value of <200 mg/dL predicts the progression to massive blood loss.
- Fibrinogen concentrate is an alternative to cryoprecipitate to replace fibrinogen when there is massive blood loss. Dosage is 70 mg/kg.

Platelets

Draft recommendations: Single donor platelets (SDPs) or apheresis platelets are collected from a single donor using as cell separators. They contain ≥3.0×10^{11} platelets (average $3.5–4.0 \times 10^{11}$) per unit in approximately 100–500 mL of plasma.

Random donor platelets (RDPs) are platelets derived from whole blood and contain ≥5.5×10^{10} platelets per bag (unit) in 40–70 mL of plasma. An adult dose consists of four to six units RDPs pooled together.

Platelets contain red cells and therefore D compatible products are preferred.

If D positive platelets are given to a D negative woman, then consider Rh D immunoglobulin.

Indications: Used to treat bleeding due to critically decreased circulating platelet counts or functionally abnormal platelets to maintain platelet count above 50,000/uL.

Response: One hour after transfusion the platelet count increment should be approximately 5,000–10,000/μL for each RDP or 10,000–60,000/μL for each SDP given.

Q3. What are the guidelines for massive transfusion?

Draft recommendations:

- *Definition:* Massive transfusion is defined as receipt of ≥10 units of packed red blood cells (RBC) in 24 hours (10/24), ≥6 units of RBC in 6 hours (6/6) and ≥5 units of RBC in 4 hours (5/4).
- *Rationale:* In a massive transfusion protocol, the blood components are organized and released by the blood bank in "packs" with specific number of components. This shortens the blood "supply time".
- Massive transfusion protocol starts with a fixed number of PRBCs, FFP, and platelets in a ratio which is generally 1:1:1.
- Requirement and components of the subsequent packs are based on the ongoing bleeding and the lab values.
- Every institution should have its MTP Protocol drafted with a clear understanding of the protocol by all those concerned.
- Activation of MTP should be done by the person who is the designated Director of the Protocol and deactivation is done by the same person once the bleeding is managed/lab values are normal.
- The transfusion of blood components is based on the laboratory results/ POC (TEG/ROTEM) findings. 2 units of FFP is transfused if INR>1.5, 1 unit of apheresis platelet is transfused if platelet count is <50,000

- 2 pools (10 units) of cryoprecipitate are transfused if fibrinogen is <200 mg/dL. Cryoprecipitate or fibrinogen concentrate is preferred over FFP when there is fibrinogen deficiency.
- Point of care instruments such as TEG and ROTEM have shown to effectively modify the requirement leading to a reduction in the overall transfusion and improving recovery rates.

Summary: Earlier, resuscitation in PPH was focused on the administration of fluids and RBCs initially to maintain hemostatic balance. FFP, cryoprecipitate, and platelets were transfused in cases where there was clinical or lab evidence of coagulopathy. Evidence has accrued to show that coagulopathy should be considered early and simultaneously with the other strategies, especially in etiologies with a higher risk of coagulopathy such as abruption or amniotic fluid embolism. There are two important goals in hemostasis. The first one is to treat hyperfibrinolysis and this is done with the administration of tranexamic acid. The second goal is equilibrium in coagulation and this is achieved with FFP, cryoprecipitate, or fibrinogen concentrate and platelets. When fibrinogen levels are less than 200 mg/dL, infusion of large volumes of FFP can further reduce fibrinogen concentration by dilution. Cryoprecipitate and fibrinogen concentrates are useful to restore equilibrium when fibrinogen levels are less than 200 mg/dL.

Viscoelastic tests like thromboelastometry (ROTEM) and thromboelastography (TEG) provide dynamic information on the speed of coagulation initiation, kinetics of clot growth, clot strength, and breakdown of clot. They can assess clinically significant low levels of fibrinogen in 10 min while lab results take much longer. Early replacement of fibrinogen is valuable in restoring hemostasis in PPH.

In the face of massive bleeding, a rapid response is the need of the hour and preparedness of the blood bank with a Massive Transfusion Protocol (MTP) facilitates a quick and effective response, thereby saving the woman and reducing the overall transfusion rate.

Q4. What is the role of recombinant factor VIIa and prothrombin complex concentrate in the hemostatic resuscitation in PPH?

Recombinant Factor VIIa (rFVIIa)

Draft recommendations:

- rFVIIa acts by boosting thrombin generation on activated platelets at endothelial damaged site leading to the formation of stable fibrin clot.
- rFVIIa should be used as an early adjuvant therapy when the standard uterotonic agents have failed to control PPH.
- Dosage 50–90 μg/kg IV bolus

European Medical Academy and Swissmedic have approved the use of recombinant factor VIIa.

Transfusion reactions: Transfusion reactions can be immediate (<24 hours) or delayed. They can range from mild to life threatening. It is important to be vigilant and recognize an adverse reaction and manage as follows.

- Transfusion should be stopped immediately
- Symptomatic treatment should be given, like antipyretics for febrile reaction ani-histamines for allergic reaction, corticosteroids if required.
- Life-threatening reactions should be evaluated clinically, investigated, and treated accordingly.
- Transfusion reaction form needs to be filled and submitted to the blood bank along with the drip set and the blood bag.

BIBLIOGRAPHY

1. Bonnet MP, Benhamou D. Management of postpartum haemorrhage. F1000Res. 2016;5:F1000 Faculty Rev-1514.
2. Coté CJ, Lerman J, Anderson BJ. A Practice of Anesthesia for Infant and Children, 6th edition. Philadelphia: Elsevier; 2019
3. Escobar M, Nassar AH, Theron G, et al. FIGO recommendations on the management of postpartum hemorrhage 2022. Int J Gynaecol Obstet. 2022;157 (Suppl 1): 3-50.
4. Hofer S, Blaha J, Collins PW, et al. Haemostatic support in postpartum haemorrhage: A review of the literature and expert opinion. Eur J Anaesthesiol. 2023;40(1):29-38.
5. Kogutt BK, Vaught AJ. Postpartum haemorrhage: Blood product management and massive transfusion. Semin Perinatol. 2019;43(1):44-50.
6. RANZCOG. (2011). Management of Postpartum Haemorrhage, Clinical Guidance Statement. [online] Available from https://ranzcog.edu.au/wp-content/uploads/Management-Postpartum-Haemorrhage.pdf. [Last accessed November, 2024]
7. RCOG. (2015). Blood transfusion in Obstetrics, RCOG Green-top Guideline No. 47. [online] Available from https://www.rcog.org.uk/guidance/browse-all-guidance/green-top-guidelines/blood-transfusions-in-obstetrics-green-top-guideline-no-47/#:~:text=The%20aim%20of%20this%20guideline,blood%20loss%20are%20also%20discussed. [Last accessed November, 2024]
8. WOMAN Trial Collaborators. Effect of early tranexamic acid administration on mortality, hysterectomy, and other morbidities in women with post-partum haemorrhage (WOMAN): an international, randomised, double-blind, placebo-controlled trial. Lancet. 2017;389(10084):2105-16.

8

CHAPTER

Minimal Surgical Management of Postpartum Hemorrhage

Nalini Mishra

Q1. What constitutes "refractory postpartum hemorrhage"? When should the second line interventions for minimal surgical management of PPH be employed?

Draft recommendations: Any postpartum hemorrhage which is not responding to the first line cause directed treatment and progressing to major PPH (blood loss >1000 mL) and is associated with worsening maternal condition (obstetric shock index >1, i.e., heart rate exceeding the systolic BP) is termed refractory PPH. Uterine atony not responding to second line uterotonic agents is also considered refractory PPH and should trigger further interventions.

Summary of evidence:

- *Defining "Refractory PPH":* WHO technical consultation in Postpartum hemorrhage care bundle (2019) defines refractory PPH as "bleeding that is unresponsive to initial treatment and that triggers an additional set of interventions , the " Response to refractory PPH bundle". The secondary analysis of the data of WHO CHAMPION trial defined refractory PPH as the one which is unresponsive to three or more uterotonics for treatment or treatment procedures.
- *Timing for second line interventions for nonsurgical management of PPH:* FIGO recommendations on the management of postpartum hemorrhage (2022) suggests that Obstetric shock index (OSI) of ≥0.9 can alert the teams regarding the need for urgent transfer. OSI of >1 increases the likelihood of blood transfusion. Green Top (RCOG) guidelines recommends further interventions along with continuing resuscitation in major PPH (blood loss >1000 ml with ongoing bleeding).

  If uterine atony does not respond to second line uterotonics, majority of guidelines of various nations (ACOG, RCOG, CNGOF, NVOG and SNLG) recommend prompt escalation of intensity of care whereas RANZCOG and DGGG do not specify the timing. In difference to these, WHO CHAMPION trial adopted the cut-off point of three uterotonics as they found that 60% of the women receiving two additional uterotonics for PPH treatment received both within a 5-minute time frame, implying that two uterotonics were often used as first-line treatment.

Maternal Health Division, Ministry of Health and Family Welfare, Government of India suggests mechanical measures for the women who do not respond to uterotonics.

Both, California Maternal Quality Care Collaborative (CMQCC) Obstetric Hemorrhage Emergency Management toolkit and Safe Motherhood Initiative (SMI) incorporate escalation of interventions in continued bleeding (>1000 but <1500 mL) after vaginal births if uterine atony is unresponsive to uterotonics OR to ≥2 uterotonics respectively. SMI recommends this even with normal vitals and lab values.

FOGSI guidelines recommended escalation to next level of interventions in cases of failure of medical management or severe or persistent PPH, while preparations for the next surgical steps are being done.

Research gap: Strong evidence regarding timing and sequence of mechanical/nonpharmacological intervention is needed.

Q2. How to proceed with nonsurgical treatment approach in a patient of refractory postpartum hemorrhage?

Draft recommendations: In refractory PPH after vaginal birth, the Bundle approach which includes the Compressive measure (aortic compression or bimanual uterine compression) Intrauterine balloon tamponade and nonpneumatic anti shock garment should be employed adopting an incremental and individualized approach. Finding and treating the cause of PPH must be done.

While choosing the second line interventions, less invasive methods should always be used first including mechanical and/or radiological measures (if available) before resorting surgical approach for management. Meanwhile continuing the resuscitative measures and uterotonics (in atonic uterus) and a second dose of tranexamic acid (after 30 minutes of the first dose) is recommended.

Summary of evidence:

- *Approach and aim:* As per WHO (2021), 10% to 20% of women are unresponsive to first response bundle. The goal of the treatment in these women is to achieve hemostasis before the patient develops coagulation problems and organ damage from under-perfusion.

  FIGO emphasizes that conservative/less invasive approaches should be tried first, rapidly moving to more invasive procedures if these do not work. Green Top Guidelines suggest a combination of pharmacological, mechanical and surgical methods directed towards the causative factor in order to arrest PPH.
- *Bundle approach for refractory PPH:* Effective nonsurgical interventions to manage refractory PPH are critical in low-resource settings where operating theatres are not always available. For patients delivering at

Algorithm chart for management of PPH after vaginal delivery

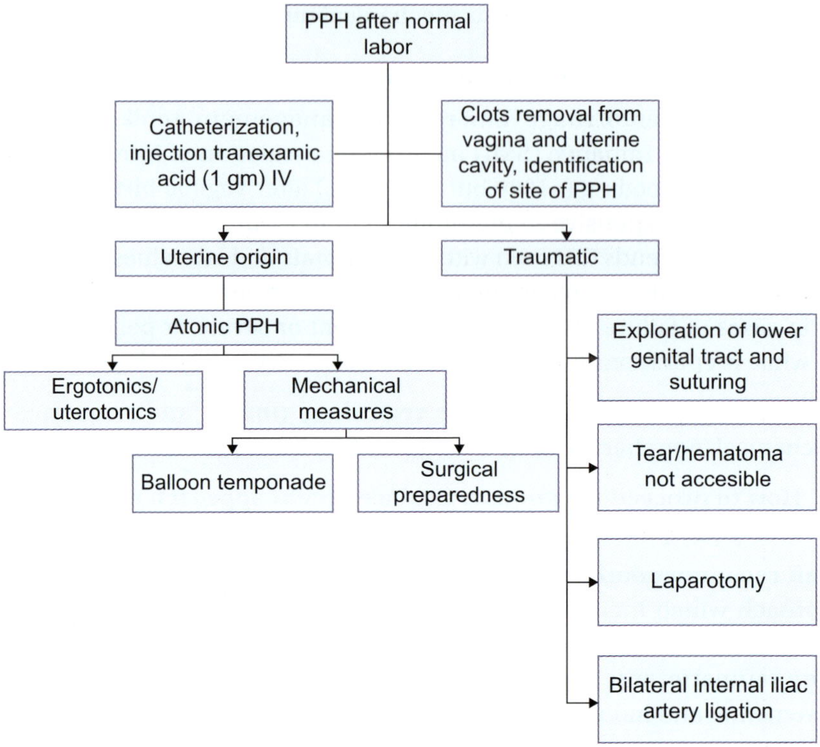

community level of healthcare system (or above), WHO recommends bimanual uterine compression, external aortic compression, the use of nonpneumatic anti-shock garment, uterine balloon tamponade (together constitute the Response to refractory PPH Bundle) and a second dose of tranexamic acid as nonsurgical interventions. This Bundle approach improves compliance with best practices of WHO recommended interventions **(Annexure 1)**.

- *Determining appropriate stepwise management:* There is neither existing data regarding the specific order in which these interventions should occur nor the comparative effectiveness of any intervention over the other.

Research gap: The specific order in which mechanical interventions should occur and the comparative effectiveness should be researched.

Q3. What is the role of Intrauterine Balloon Tamponade (IBT) device in refractory PPH?

Draft recommendations: Uterine balloon tamponade is recommended in cases of refractory PPH as a component of "response to refractory PPH bundle" in all women delivering at community level of healthcare or above

Algorithm chart for management of PPH in cesarean section

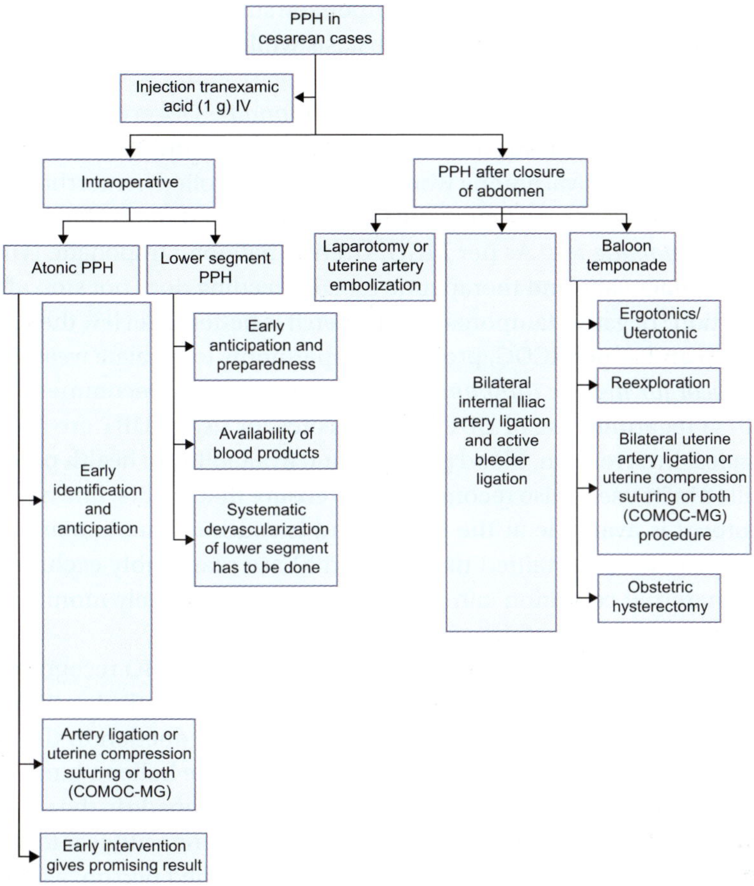

and due to uterine atony. It should be employed early before the advanced stages of shock. Intrauterine balloon tamponade device can be any available device (commercially available one or prepared at the point of care from available material at low resource settings e.g. condom balloon tamponade device). Uterine balloon tamponade should be performed by a competent health care provider trained and skilled in the management of PPH. Other causes of PPH should be reasonably excluded.

Summary of evidence:

- *Recommendation base for uterine balloon tamponade:* In case of refractory PPH due to uterine atony, once additional/other sources of PPH have been excluded, mechanical tamponade is recommended by the WHO, FIGO, Govt of India, FOGSI, ACOG, RCOG, SOGC, Australian & New Zealand (RANZCOG), French (CNGOF), Netherlands (NVOG) SMI and CMQCC.

The German guidelines (DGGG) stress not to rule out other therapeutic options, suggesting that uterine tamponade should be seen as a 'bridging' measure to accomplish brief hemostasis while preparing the patient for more invasive definite interventions.

- *The effectiveness of uterine balloon tamponade:* Observational studies have reported UBT success rates between 83% and 95% overall with nearly 100% survival among women with uncontrolled hemorrhage when a UBT device is placed before the onset of advanced shock (FIGO 2022).
- *The tamponade test:* As per FIGO, Uterine balloon tamponade (UBT) is both a diagnostic and therapeutic tool. If bleeding does not stop after its insertion (negative tamponade test) then it is better to review the etiology of PPH and as per RCOG, proceed to laparotomy to escalate treatment.
- *Protocol for uterine tamponade:* According to WHO recommendations (2021) regarding use of UBT, prerequisites for use of UBT are access to surgical intervention, blood products and availability of health personnel skilled in its use. It also recommends to ensure that the first line treatment protocol is available at the facility and is routinely implemented. The other causes of (retained tissue, trauma) are reasonably excluded and the maternal condition can be regularly and adequately monitored for prompt recognition of deterioration if any.

  FIGO guideline the above protocol in terms that WHO recognizes that conditions may not be operationalized across all clinical settings and that observational studies suggest a substantial reduction in the risk of maternal morbidity and mortality following uterine balloon tamponade. FIGO therefore recommends uterine balloon tamponade in the context of refractory PPH as it has proven to be an effective nonsurgical technique so that when employed rapidly by a properly trained person, as the only prerequisite for its use, it can potentially improve survival in women with PPH.
- *Available UBT devices and their comparative effectiveness:*
  - *Commercially available devices (need procurement):* Bakri balloon®, BT-Cath® and EBB® (have a central drainage port), ESM-UBT, Ellavi UBT and Zukovski
  - *Devices assembled at the point of care using components available in the facility:* Condom balloon tamponade (CBT), e.g., easy balloon **(Annexure 2A)**, Glove balloon tamponade, improvised CBT, e.g., CG balloon which has a central drainage port **(Annexure 2B)**

  FIGO quotes "the success rates of condom UBT devices appear to be comparable to those of commercial device".

Research gap: Insufficient evidence from RCTs, strong need for further research is in low-resource settings regarding which preconditions are the most important to obtain clinical benefits from UBT.

Q4. Which temporizing mechanical measures yield the best results in postpartum hemorrhage while awaiting definitive interventions?

Draft recommendations: Temporizing mechanical measures such as compressions either manual (external aortic or bimanual uterine compression) or with devices like Non pneumatic antishock garment (NASG) are recommended in cases of refractory PPH as a component of "Response to refractory PPH Bundle" while awaiting definitive intervention for hemostasis which are cause directed or for allowing blood transfusions or transfer to a higher facility.

NASG is a low technology, affordable, light weight first-aid lower body compression device for the stabilization of women having major PPH. It allows an easy access to vagina and perineum and thereby facilitate surgical interventions through vaginal route.

Summary of evidence:

- *Recommendations about compressions:* The WHO recommended "Bundle approach to refractory PPH" includes external aortic compression, bimanual uterine compression, IBT and Non pneumatic antishock garment (NASG).This applies to vaginal deliveries whereas a post caesarean bleeding may require a modified approach. ACOG and CMQCC recommend manual compression in unresponsive bleeding. RCOG recommends compression of the aorta as a temporary but effective measure to allow time for resuscitation to catch up with the volume replacement and the appropriate surgical support to arrive **(Annexure 1)**.
- *NASG:* FIGO (2022) recommends the use of the nonpneumatic anti-shock garment for hypovolemic shock secondary to obstetric hemorrhage showing signs of shock/hemodynamic instability, at the primary healthcare level or if transport to higher facility is necessary: EBL 500 ml, SBP <100 mm Hg, pulse >100 bpm; at high-level facilities: EBL >1000 ml, SBP < 90 mm Hg, pulse > 110 bpm (or per facility protocols) and is subject to modifications Depending on capacity of facility and staff, the NASG could also be applied as first-line , first aid.

Use of the NASG combined with standard PPH care reduces both maternal mortality by 48% with a relative risk of 0.52 (95% CI, 0.36–0.77) and a 68% reduction in combined adverse outcomes, mortality, and severe morbidities (RR 0.31; 95%CI, 0.17–0.59). Furthermore, no adverse effects have been documented with correct implementation of the NASG and no increase in shock-related organ dysfunction adverse effects have been noted. Currently, there are no absolute medical contraindications for NASG use. In severe hemorrhage, benefits are thought to outweigh any potential harm.

Q5. Role of selective arterial embolization in the treatment of PPH?

Draft recommendations: Selective arterial embolization (UAE) can be considered in a woman having refractory PPH but is hemodynamically stable and appear to have persistent slow bleeding despite less invasive therapeutic measures and if the resources for intervention radiology are available. UAE is NOT recommended for brisk ongoing bleeding that would not allow time to accomplish embolization.

Pelvic arteries catheterization with deflated endovascular balloon may be considered in patients with a preexisting diagnosis of placenta accreta syndrome (abnormally invasive placenta) with an intention to inflate the balloon after delivery of the baby. The endovascular occlusion may also helpful in secondary PPH as it hastens the placental necrosis in cases where placenta is left in situ.

Summary of evidence:

- *Recommendations:* Recommended by WHO (2012), if other measures have failed and the necessary resources are available. Other guidelines also recommend it when second-line uterotonics fail. A recent systematic review and a meta-analysis concluded that UAE has beneficial effects on refractory PPH. UAE significantly reduced blood loss with shortened operating time, lower use of RBC units and length of stay compared with hysterectomy but no difference between the UAE group and hysterectomy group in hemostatic effective rate or mortality.
- *Limits of recommendation:* WHO "PPH Bundle" (2019) has excluded arterial embolization from bundles as it is not feasible in most settings. German guideline recommends transcatheter arterial embolization as a last resort after surgical treatment has been exhausted. The UK guideline underlines the logistical limits that 'the equipment or an interventional radiologist may not be available".

  International Society for PAS (IS-PAS) could not recommend routine use of prophylactic pelvic arterial balloon catheters for all cases of suspected AIP in view of a systematic review looking at endovascular interventional modalities for hemorrhage control in AIP due to low quality cohort and significant heterogeneity.
- *Comparative effectiveness of UAE versus other non-pharmacologic measures:* A recent meta-analysis of comparative effectiveness of non-pharmacologic managements on postpartum hemorrhage concluded that for the quick treatment of postpartum bleeding, balloon tamponade is the best method for uncontrolled postpartum bleeding with pharmacologic treatment, followed by uterine artery embolization and surgical procedures. Green Top Guidelines opine that UBT is more appropriate where the equipment or an interventional radiologist may not be available.

- *Typical order of intervention after vaginal delivery if the facility for UAE exists:* As per CMQCC toolkit, selective embolization should typically follow UBT and precede surgical recourse. FIGO (2022) recommends that if choice between UAE and uterine artery ligation is available, embolization is preferred as it obviates laparotomy. Ligation can be attempted subsequently if embolization is unsuccessful. In contrast, after an unsuccessful uterine artery ligation, embolization may be extremely difficult or even impossible leaving hysterectomy as the only remaining option. Both procedures have reported success rates of greater than 90%. Some cases may require hysterectomy because of failure of embolization.
- *Role of UAE in secondary bleeding:* UAE has shown to be effective in controlling secondary bleeding and the placenta was found to gradually decrease in size in all patients. UAE plays an important role in managing these patients because it is effective at reducing uteroplacental blood flow to further induce thrombosis of the intervillous space and to achieve necrosis of the retained placental tissue.

  Complications of pelvic arterial embolization: In traumatic PPH and post hysterectomy hemoperitoneum

  The complications of pelvic embolization for PPH may occur in 8.7% cases. The most common complication is low-grade fever. Less common complications are pelvic infection, groin hematoma, iliac artery perforation, transient buttock ischemia, transient foot ischemia, bladder gangrene, dissection of the uterine arteries, hematoma at the puncture site, paresthesia and lower limb edema. As per a recent systemic review, the procedure may be associated with increased risk of PPH and placenta accrete spectrum in subsequent pregnancies.

Research gap: There is little randomized trial evidence regarding efficacy and requires further research.

Q6. What is the evidence in support of emerging techniques in mechanical/ nonpharmacological management of PPH?

Draft recommendations: The emerging techniques are spread across a wide range of publications and have not been summarized as evidence. There is a lack of robust evidence of effectiveness of most individual methods but at the same time all innovative methods provide the clinicians with something to implement as a last resort in cases of refractory PPH.

Summary of evidence:

- *Emerging techniques of uterine suction tamponade:* This is an alternative approach to uterine tamponade based upon uterine contraction and retraction. The purpose- designed Jada system (AlydiaHealth) has been approved by the Federal Drug Administration in USA. Some improvised suction devices like Vacuum Suction cannula are also used.

Annexure 1

Mechanical Methods for Refractory Postpartum Hemorrhage: Temporizing Measures

Bimanual Uterine (Fig. 1): A Temporary Measure

- Wear sterile gloves preferably elbow length.
- One hand is placed on the fundus.
- Under all aseptic precautions, the second hand is lubricated and placed anterior to the cervix.
- The abdominal hand is now placed on the posterior aspect of the fundus.

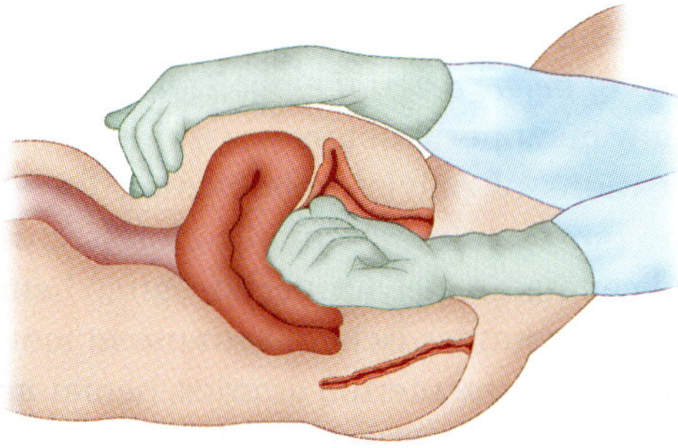

Fig. 1: Bimanual compression.

Manual Aortic Compression (Fig. 2): A Temporary Measure

- Stand on the side of woman.
- Place your fist just above and to the left side of the umbilicus, thumb should be outside the fist.

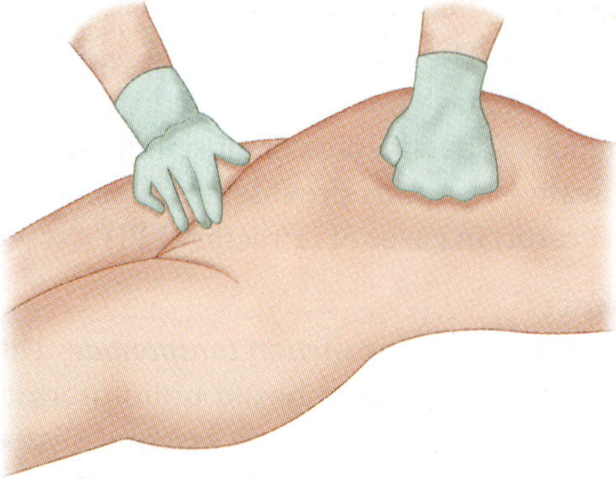

Fig. 2: Abdominal aortic compression.

- If needed, stand on a raised platform and then lean over the woman so that the aorta can be felt against your knuckles.
- Feel for femoral pulse.
- Apply pressure with the flat of your fist over the aorta, keep your elbow joint fully extended so as to exert sufficient pressure until femoral pulse is not felt.
- Continue pressure until further help arrives/definitive measures are in place.

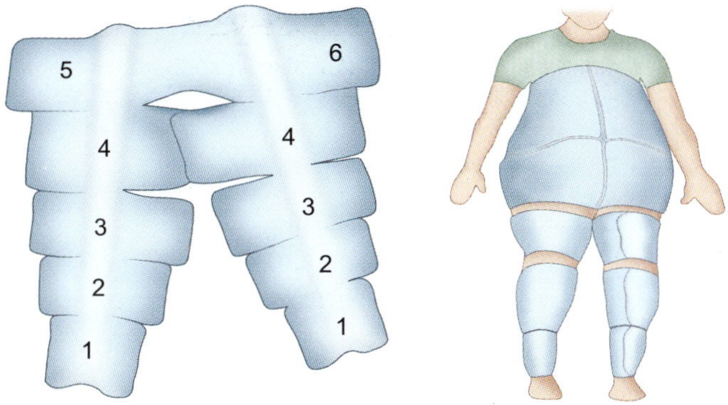

Fig. 3: Nonpneumatic antishock garment (NASG).

First-aid device when access to the definitive treatment is awaited particularly in women with PPH and shock who need transfer to higher-level facilities.

Steps:

- Put an indwelling catheter in bladder.
- Spread NASG on the bed under the woman with the upper edge of NASG at the level of lowest rib of the woman **(Fig. 3)**.
- Start fastening the segments enclosing ankle, thigh, calves, pelvis, and abdomen respectively as per the numbers indicated on the same. It is done with the help of Velcro fastenings till a distinct snap is heard indicating the optimal tightening of the garment.
- A small foam ball in the abdominal segment applies pressure directly over the uterus when the abdominal segment is closed.
- Keep the knee joints free.
- Ensure that the woman is breathing comfortably.
- The NASG can remain in place during any vaginal procedure and if surgical recourse is required, the abdominal segment can be opened for the duration of surgery and refasten.
- Removal of the NASG is done only when the cause-directed treatment of PPH is done successfully and the woman has been hemodynamically stable for at least 2 hours, and blood loss is <50 mL/h.

- Removal begins at the ankles and proceeds slowly, waiting 15 minutes between opening each segment, and taking vital signs (blood pressure and pulse) before opening the next segment. If pulse rate increases >20 BPM or BP falls by 20 mm Hg, reapply segment.
- Wash NASG with running water followed by disinfection. Air dry it and keep it folded in a transparent plastic bag.

Annexure 2

Condom Balloon Tamponade Devices

2A: *Condom balloon tamponade device (Easy):* Easiest way to assemble condom balloon tamponade.

Material needed: Condom, Foley's catheter (any available size), IV set, and saline

Steps ***(Figs. 1A to D)****:*

A. Cut two rings of 1 millimeter width from the drainage port of Foley's catheter. Unfold the condom over the proximal one-third of the Foley's catheter.
B. Secure the condom to the catheter with the help of the one of the rings prepared (as step 1A) at the distance of 1–2 cm from the rim of the condom by encircling twice over it.
C. The device (CBT) is then dipped in antiseptic solution for at least 3 minutes. In the meantime, the woman is put in lithotomy position and anterior lip of cervix is grasped with sponge holding forceps. CBT is now inserted into the uterine cavity by holding it between two fingers. Distal end of the catheter is connected to the infusion set of normal saline. The device is now inflated till either the bleeding stops or an amount of 500 mL is reached.
D. After ensuring hemostasis, the lower end of CBT device is occluded with the other ring prepared in step (A) by encircling it around the folded distal end thrice. Pack the vagina to keep CBT in place.

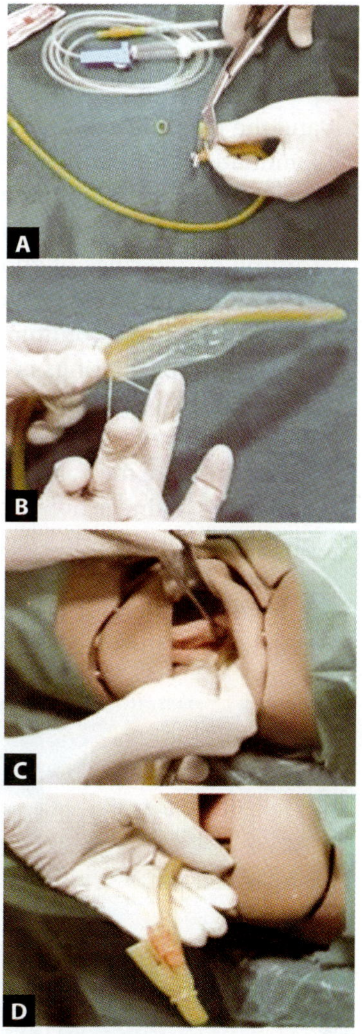

Figs. 1A to D

Postplacement care: Catheterize the bladder, mark the boundaries of the uterus on abdomen, start oxytocin 10 U in 500 mL NS @40 drops/min for 4–6 hours. Give antibiotics and monitor closely.

Removal of CBT: 6–24 hours later in routine hours. Simply unfold the lower end and the saline drains away, wait for 30 minutes, monitor closely, reinflate if bleeding recurs.

2B: CG Balloon: Modified condom balloon tamponade device with a central drainage port

Material required: Foley's catheter (20–24 Fr), condom, scissors, two 20-mL syringes, and saline (500 mL)

Steps ***(Figs. 2A to F)****:*

A. Air (20 cc) is introduced into the bulb of the catheter which is then punctured with scissors and the bulb is then incised circumferentially and the flaps are everted up and down so that the hole on the shaft used for inflating the bulb is well exposed.
B. Balloon is made by unfolding of condom over proximal one-third of the catheter keeping the tip of the catheter in the tip of the condom.
C. Cutting of two rings of approximately 1 mm in width is done from the distal end of the drainage tube of Foley's catheter.
D. Double secure the condom over the catheter using the rings obtained by step C, first of the rings is applied at the niche produced by excision of the bulb (the so-called neck) encircling around twice like a rubber band. The second one is applied 1 cm from the rim of condom.
E. Excise the tip of the Foley's catheter and condom together at the middle of the Foley's drainage hole. This creates the drainage hole at the top to drain blood from the uterine cavity. The device is then dipped in antiseptic solution for at least 3 minutes. Woman is put in lithotomy position and anterior lip of cervix is grasped with sponge holding forceps. Device is inserted into the uterine cavity by holding it between two fingers. Vagina

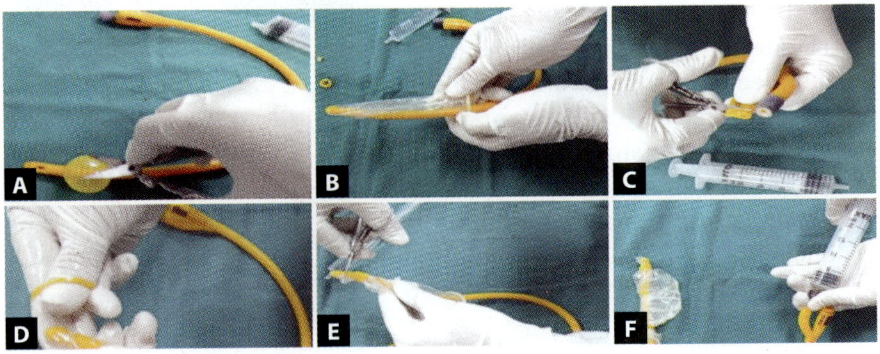

Figs. 2A to F

is now packed with gauze/dressing pads to prevent expulsion of balloon during inflation. The drainage port is connected to a collecting bag for measuring the ongoing blood loss.

F. Fill the balloon is filled with saline (maximum 500 mL) through the bulb-inflation port of the catheter using syringes in repetitive manner until the bleeding is controlled (bleeding <1 mL/min as assessed at the drainage port)

Postplacement care: Catheterize the bladder, mark the boundaries of the uterus on abdomen, start oxytocin 10 U in 500 mL NS @40 drops/min for 4–6 hours, give antibiotics and monitor closely.

Removal: 6–24 hours later by aspirating saline back from through bulb inflation port. Wait for half an hour, reinflate if bleeding recurs.

BIBLIOGRAPHY

1. ACOG Practice Bulletin No. 183 summary: postpartum hemorrhage. Obstet Gynecol. 2017;130(4):923-5.
2. California Maternal quality Care Collaborative (CMQCC). (2015). Obstetric Hemorrhage Toolkit. version 2. [online] Available from https://www.cmqcc.org/resources-tool-kits/toolkits/ob-hemorrhage-toolkit [Last accessed November, 2024].
3. De Vries PLM, Deneux-Tharaux C, Baud D, et al. Postpartum haemorrhage in high- resource settings: Variations in clinical management and future research directions based on a comparative study of national guidelines. BJOG. 2023; 130(13):1639-52.
4. DHEERA. (2022). FOGSI Updated Guidelines for PPH Prevention and Management. [online] Available from. https://www.fogsi.org/wp-content/uploads/tog/pph-prevention-and-management-updated-sept-2022.pdf [Last accessed November, 2024].
5. Escobar M, Nassar AH, Theron G, et al. FIGO recommendations on the management of postpartum hemorrhage 2022. Int J Gynaecol Obstet. 2022;157 (Suppl 1): 3-50.
6. Fernandez MG, Coutinho de Carvalho SF, Martins BA, et al. Uterine Artery Embolization Versus Hysterectomy in Postpartum Hemorrhage: A Systematic Review With Meta-Analysis. J Endovasc Ther. 2024:15266028241252730.
7. Goffman D, Ananth CV, Fleischer A, et al; Safe Motherhood Initiative Obstetric Hemorrhage Work Group. The new york state safe motherhood initiative: early impact of obstetric hemorrhage bundle implementation. Am J Perinatol. 2019;36(13):1344-50.
8. Hofmeyr. Novel concepts and improvisation for treating postpartum haemorrhage: a narrative review of emerging techniques. Reprod Health. 2023; 20:116.
9. IS-AIP, Collins SL, Alemdar B, et al. Evidence-based guidelines for the management of abnormally invasive placenta: Recommendations from the International Society for Abnormally Invasive Placenta. Am J Obstet Gynecol. 2019;220(6):511-26.

10. Jiang L, Wang X. A new non-invasive procedure for refractory PPH after vaginal delivery and caesarean section. J Obstet Gynaecol. 2021;41(5):791-6.
11. Kellie FJ, Wandabwa JN, Mousa HA, et al. Mechanical and surgical interventions for treating primary postpartum haemorrhage. Cochrane Database Syst Rev. 2020;7(7):CD013663.
12. Lee KJ, Hong K, Hwang H, et al. Perspective of the comparative effectiveness of non-pharmacologic managements on postpartum hemorrhage meta-analysis. Obstet Gynecol Sci. 2020;63(5):605-14.
13. Liu LY, Nathan L, Sheen JJ, et al. Review of Current Insights and Therapeutic Approaches for the Treatment of Refractory Postpartum Hemorrhage. Int J Womens Health. 2023;15:905-26.
14. Liu Z, Wang Y, Yan J, et al. Uterine artery embolization versus hysterectomy in the treatment of refractory postpartum hemorrhage: a systematic review and meta-analysis. J Matern Fetal Neonatal Med. 2020;33(4):693-705.
15. Maternal Health Division, Ministry of Health and Family Welfare, Government of India. (2015). Guidance Note on Prevention and Management of Postpartum Haemorrhage. [online] Available from https://nhm.gov.in/images/pdf/programmes/maternal-health/guidelines/Guidance_Note_on_Prevention_&_Management_of_Postpartum_Haemorrhage.pdf [Last accessed November, 2024].
16. Matsuzaki S, Lee M, Nagase Y, et al. A systematic review and meta-analysis of obstetric and maternal outcomes after prior uterine artery embolization. Sci Rep. 2021;11(1):16914.
17. Mavrides EAS, Chandraharan E, Collins P, et al. Prevention and management of post-partum haemorrhage: green-top guideline No 52. BJOG. 2017;124: e106-49.
18. Mishra N, Gulabani K, Agrawal S, et al. Efficacy and Feasibility of Chhattisgarh Balloon and Conventional Condom Balloon Tamponade: A 2-Year Prospective Study. J Obstet Gynaecol India. 2019;69(Suppl 2):133-41.
19. Ordoñez CA, Manzano-Nunez R, Parra MW, et al. Prophylactic use of resuscitative endovascular balloon occlusion of the aorta in women with abnormal placentation: a systematic review, meta-analysis, and case series. J Trauma Acute Care Surg. 2018;84(5):809-18.
20. Postpartum hemorrhage care bundles to improve adherence to guidelines: A WHO technical consultation. Int J Gynecol Obstet. 2018;143(Suppl 3):973.
21. Ramanathan A, Eckardt MJ, Nelson BD, et al Safety of a condom uterine balloon tamponade (ESM-UBT) device for uncontrolled primary postpartum hemorrhage among facilities in Kenya and Sierra Leone. BMC Pregnancy Childbirth. 2018;18:168.
22. Shahin Y, Pang CL. Endovascular interventional modalities for haemorrhage control in abnormal placental implantation deliveries: a systematic review and meta-analysis. Eur Radiol 2018;28(7):2713-26.
23. Tindell K, Garfinkel R, Abu-Haydar E, et al. Uterine balloon tamponade 1435 for the treatment of postpartum haemorrhage in resource-poor settings: a systematic review. BJOG. 2013;120:5-14.
24. WHO. WHO recommendation on uterine balloon tamponade for the treatment of postpartum haemorrhage. Geneva: World Health Organization; 2021.
25. Widmer M, Piaggio G, Hofmeyr GJ, et al. Maternal characteristics and causes associated with refractory postpartum haemorrhage after vaginal birth: a secondary analysis of the WHO CHAMPION trial data. BJOG. 2020;127: 628-34.

CHAPTER 9

Surgical Management of Postpartum Hemorrhage

Shashi L Kabra Maheshwari, T Chitra, Ashis K Mukhopadhyay

PELVIC VASCULATURE LIGATION

Bilateral Uterine Artery Ligature

Background

The first cases of bilateral uterine artery ligature (BUAL) were published by Waters in 1952 and O'Leary in 1966. It is an easy, fast, and safe procedure to stop bleeding located in body of uterus during a laparotomy. Uterine arteries are responsible for nearly 90% of irrigation of uterine body, and so it may be a successful procedure for controlling bleeding in this area. However, it is not effective in bleeding from lower uterine segment, cervix and paracolpos **(Flowchart 1)**.

Flowchart 1: Steps of sequential surgical management of refractory postpartum hemorrhage (PPH).

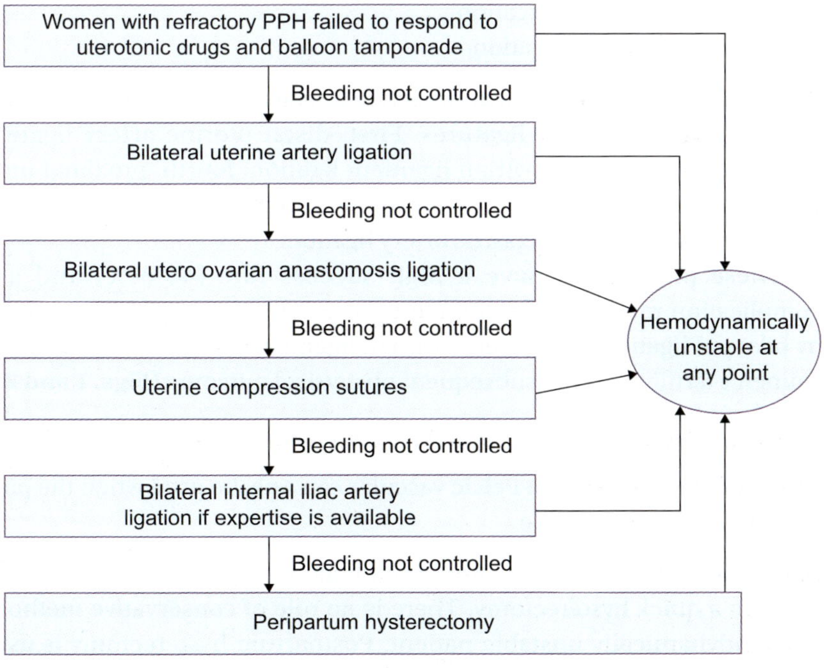

Q1. What is Stepwise uterine devascularization and in which stage of refractory PPH, are these procedures most helpful?

Draft recommendations: Bilateral Uterine artery ligation (BUAL) and utero ovarian anastomosis ligation are an important and useful management modality in a refractory case of PPH when Medical, mechanical, and non-surgical treatment and compression sutures have failed in controlling bleeding. The success rate is 40 -90%. It is a type of uterus-preserving surgery and is to be done only when the patient is hemodynamically stable. It is an essential skill for a gynecologist.

Discussion: Since its description for the treatment of PPH in 1960, uterine artery ligation has gained popularity as one of the most straightforward and quick surgical methods for retaining fertility. It is a successful management technique for stopping bleeding, with success rates between 42% and 88%.

FIGO recommends uterine artery ligation as one of the options to rapidly control PPH when medical, nonsurgical approaches and compression sutures fail.

Q2. What are the different methods of pelvic vascular ligation in PPH?

Draft recommendations:

- Bilateral uterine artery ligation
- Upper and lower uterine artery ligation
- Utero-ovarian artery ligation
- Internal iliac artery ligation

Discussion: The methodical approach delineated by comprises a sequential progression of vascular ligatures. First, distal uterine artery ligation is performed; next, utero-ovarian ligament ligation; fourth, proximal uterine artery ligation is performed to control persistent bleeding; and, lastly, the fifth and final step is hypogastric artery ligation.

These procedures have a high success rate (45-80%) and a low complication rate. Ligation of the uterine arteries, whether or not followed by bilateral ligation of the utero-ovarian ligaments, does not seem to impair women's fertility or their subsequent obstetrical outcome **(Figs. 1 and 2)**.

Q3. What is the prerequisite for the use of this procedure?

Draft recommendations: Pelvic vascular can only be used when the patient is hemodynamically stable.

Discussion: If the patient is not hemodynamically stable, then we should perform a quick hysterectomy. There is no role of conservative methods in a hemodynamically unstable patient. Postpartum hysterectomy is usually indicated when all conservative measures have failed (or are not indicated)

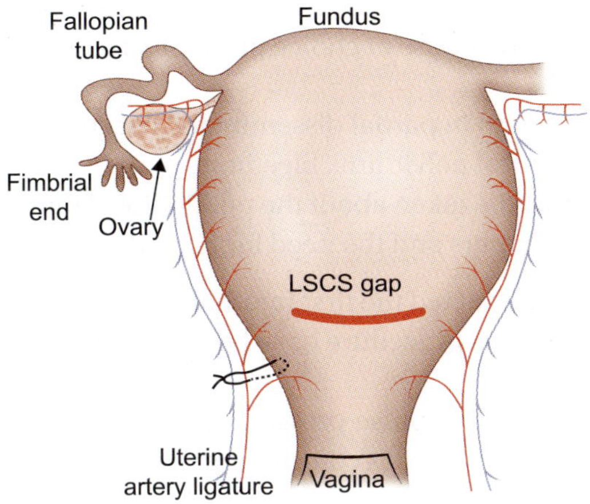

Fig. 1: Distal (lower) uterine artery ligation.

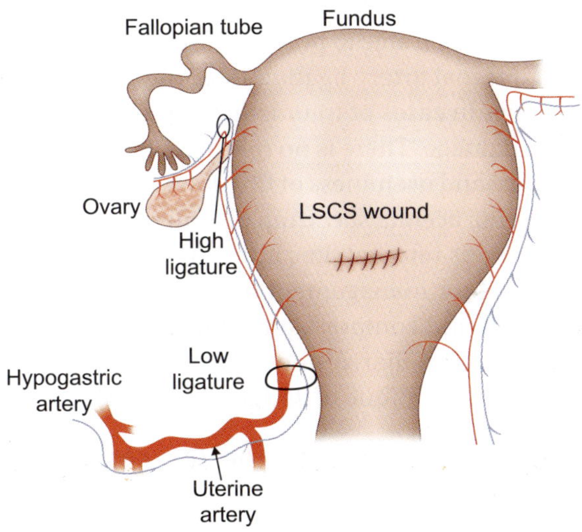

Fig. 2: Utero-ovarian artery anastomosis ligation.

to achieve bleeding control. However, when it is indicated, it should be performed as early as possible, to avoid the installation of coagulopathy.

Q4. What is the role of internal iliac artery ligation (IIAL) in atonic and traumatic PPH? What consent needs to be taken before performing this procedure?

Draft recommendations: Bilateral Internal iliac artery ligation (BIIAL) is a life-saving surgery for both traumatic and atonic postpartum hemorrhage

BIIAL blocks supply to the uterine artery which is the major blood supply to the uterus. It is the procedure of choice in a case of a retracted uterine artery in a traumatic PPH.

BIIAL is also helpful in partial disseminated coagulopathy and even after hysterectomy to control pelvic area bleeding.

Consent needs to be taken about the possibility of injury to nearby major veins, arteries and ureters and the need for ICU admission.

Discussion: Kelly conducted the first Internal iliac artery ligation in 1894.

Success rates for this procedure have been reported to range from 40% to 100%.

Bilateral IIAl decreases pulse pressure by 85 %, converts arterial flow to venous flow, and thus facilitates coagulation. Pelvic blood flow is reduced to half.

Despite being a quick and effective method of controlling bleeding, this technique is still rarely used due to the reasonable fear of harming the ureters and internal and external iliac arteries. It should only be taken into consideration if skilled pelvic surgeons are available. In the case of uterine atony, internal iliac artery ligation may be able to prevent the need for a hysterectomy.

In addition, internal artery ligation frees the operating field and makes hysterectomy easier in cases of traumatic PPH, such as uterine rupture and extensive genital damage. There is no role of unilateral internal iliac ligation.

The importance and usefulness of IIAL have increased with the increased incidence of Placenta accreta spectrum disorder, in recent years.

FIGO recommends internal iliac artery ligation as one of the options to rapidly control PPH for management of PPH when medical, and minimal surgical approaches and compression sutures fail. FIGO also recommends that all obstetricians familiarize themselves with the internal iliac artery location and with the technique of its ligation **(Fig. 3)**.

Q5. What are important technical errors that can happen with IIAL and how to prevent these?

Draft recommendations:

- One may injure great vessels while opening the retroperitoneum and dissection of the retroperitoneum.
    - Opening the retroperitoneum under a clear vision and gradually saving the underlying structure is advisable.
    - Only finger dissection is recommended once the retroperitoneum is opened as this safeguard will prevent inadvertent injury to common iliac, external iliac, internal iliac arteries, and veins.
- The movement of passing the right-angle forceps (Mixter) in between the Internal iliac artery and vein should always be from lateral to medial on both sides. This will prevent injury to the External iliac vein.

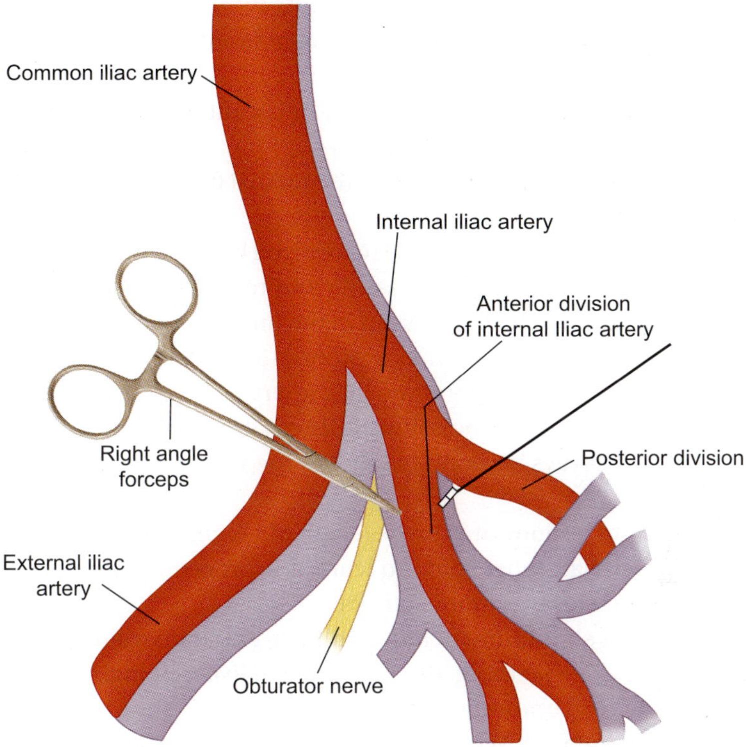

Fig. 3: Ligation of the anterior division on the Internal iliac artery.

Discussion: The following complications could arise from the ligation of an IIA:

Ligation or laceration of the external iliac artery:

Technical error—failure to localize the external iliac artery by noticing a change in pulse in the femoral artery when the External iliac artery is pressed.

Ligation or laceration of the ureter:

Technical error: Failure to open the anterior leaf of the broad ligament in the correct direction. The direction of dissection should be towards the lateral pelvic wall and parallel to the infundibulopelvic ligament.

Failure to identify ureter in the medial flap.

Injury to Externa and internal iliac vein:

Technical error: Failure to pass the ligature passer or Mixter forceps from lateral to medial direction hits the external iliac vein.

Improper Dissection technique between artery and vein leads to injury to the vein.

Q6. Recommendations for mastering this technique.

Draft recommendations: Obstetricians must familiarize themselves with the anatomy and relations of IIAL.

Always recognize the inverted Y, i.e., bifurcation of the common iliac artery into external and internal iliac artery.

The ureter should always be seen in the medial flap and pushed medially in the medial flap.

The external iliac artery should be recognized by observing changes in the distal pulse by an assistant after pressing and reappearance after releasing pressure. There is no such change seen in the Internal iliac artery.

Recognize the site of ligation as a point 4–5 cm below the origin of the internal iliac artery from the common iliac artery.

Dissection of the sheath enclosing the Internal iliac artery and the internal iliac vein should always be done parallel to the vessel. This will help avoid vein injury.

Dissection is to be done only in the length of 1-2 cm of arterial length only.

Every Obstetrician must begin to learn this procedure and must utilize this procedure in relevant circumstances.

Teaching IIAL should be included in post-graduate training programs (regular classes, video learning, discussions, and live training.

The practice of opening the retroperitoneum should be done in gynecological surgeries. While performing a hysterectomy, the surgeon should practice opening the retroperitoneum routinely and should practice visualizing the ureter in the medial flap.

Discussion: The primary circulatory supply for the visceral components of the pelvis is the internal iliac artery. To stop significant pelvic hemorrhage, all pelvic surgeons need to be familiar with the anatomic features and fundamentals of internal iliac artery ligation.

FIGO also recommends that all obstetricians familiarize themselves with the internal iliac artery location and with the technique of its ligation.

COMPRESSION SUTURES

Q7. What is effectiveness of compression sutures in the management of atonic PPH?

Draft recommendations: When medical management and uterotonics fail to control bleeding, surgical interventions such as compression sutures become essential. The most widely studied and utilized technique, the B-Lynch suture has demonstrated a high success rate of over 90% in stopping hemorrhage and preserving the uterus. Hemostatic suture techniques are effective in controlling severe PPH and in reducing the need for hysterectomy.

FIGO recommends compression sutures as one of the options to control PPH when medical and nonsurgical treatment modalities fail.

Laminated diagram of the brace suture technique should be kept in theatre.

The hemostatic suturing technique is a quick, effective, and conservative second-line method for controlling uterine bleeding due to atony, suitable after both cesarean and vaginal deliveries when initial management fails. Compression sutures can be applied to slow the bleeding, stabilize the patient, avoid the need for a hysterectomy, and ultimately reduce maternal morbidity and mortality. The most used compression suture techniques for PPH are B-Lynch, Hayman, and Pereira. Christopher B-Lynch was the first to highlight this technique of Compression sutures.

In the original studies for B-Lynch, Hayman, and Pereira, success rates were reported as 100% (5/5 for B-Lynch, 3/3 for Hayman, and 7/7 for Pereira). A systematic review reported an overall success rate of 91.7% for compression sutures ranging from 76% to 100% across 9 summarized original articles, though reliable data is lacking. To date, no randomized controlled trials (RCTs) or controlled trials have been conducted to determine which uterine compression suture is the most effective for achieving hemostasis. A prospective population based UK study reported a lower success rate than other reports, but compression sutures still achieved an overall success rate of 75%.

Using a compression suture within one hour after delivery resulted in a higher success rate of 84%. A delay of two to six hours from delivery to the application of a uterine compression suture was independently associated with a fourfold increase in the risk of hysterectomy. In a comprehensive British population-based study, Kayem et al., discovered that the timing of compression suture application significantly affected their success rate. Sutures applied within the first hour post-delivery achieved an 84% success rate, whereas a delay of 2 to 6 hours reduced the success rate to 58%.

Q8. What is the effectiveness of uterine compression sutures with additional hemostatic procedures for the management of postpartum hemorrhage?

Draft recommendations: The B-Lynch suture, either in isolation or combined with other techniques, proves to be a straightforward and efficacious strategy for controlling atonic PPH. Compression sutures along with uterine artery ligation is one of the options to rapidly control PPH when medical, nonsurgical approaches.

Placing a UBT after application of uterine compression sutures requires control of the amount of pressure exerted in the uterus to prevent uterine necrosis.

In the study by Kaya et al., Bakri balloon tamponade, a less invasive uterine-preserving method, was compared with the B-Lynch compression suture. Their prospective study found similar success rates, mean time to bleeding control, estimated blood loss, and numbers of transfused packed red blood cells for both methods. While uterine necrosis can occur with compression sutures alone, the risk understandably increases with the additional pressure exerted by the UBT.

A Systematic review of data from various study groups, indicates that uterine artery occlusion (UAL) is a safe and effective intervention for managing severe postpartum hemorrhage (PPH). In a prospective comparative controlled studies comparing B-Lynch with UAL, the authors did not find any significant difference between both the groups in reducing blood loss after a cesarean section. The total blood loss within 6 hours postoperatively for the study groups was significantly lower (251.02±21.83 ml and 246.00±21.39 ml) compared to the control group (332.62±18.87 ml) ($p < 0.001$)

Q9. What are the complications of the compression sutures?

Draft recommendations: B-lynch and Hayman compression sutures are associated with a low complication rate compared to CHO sutures.

To best of our Knowledge, there have been no reports of maternal mortality but however morbidity events has been documented, including uterine necrosis, pyometra, and uterine synechiae. While specific data are lacking, the Cho suture appears to be linked to complications more frequently than other sutures. This is likely because these complications may arise from "compression tightness" and "uterine penetration." Although the Cho suture provides effective hemostasis, it can also cause complications related to the compression.

Q10. Which suture material and needle is best for compression sutures?

Draft recommendations: Monocryl is ideal suture material for uterine compression which is firm and mono filamentary with no adverse effects. Dedicated curved needle with customized sizable and a straight super blunt straight needle is ideal. Whether dedicated needles can improve the uterine preservation rate remains unclear.

Various suture materials have been utilized in uterine compression sutures, including chromic catgut, polyglycolic acid (PGA), polyglactin 910 (Vicryl), polydioxanone (PDS), monofilament polypropylene (Prolene), and poliglecaprone 25 (Monocryl). The ideal suture material for uterine compression should be firm and monofilamentary to minimize damage to the uterine wall, rapidly absorbable to reduce the risk of bowel entrapment and intrauterine adhesions, and mounted on a large curved needle to facilitate easy operation. The Monocryl absorption profile is 60%, 20%, and 0% of the original strength at 7, 14, and 21 days.

In a systematic review on the needle and suture types for uterine compression sutures involving 76 studies, where suture sizes 0, 1, and 2 were used in 6, 44, and 32 articles, respectively found about 80% of previous articles used Catgut and Polyglactin 910 sutures. They found that uterine preservation rate was significantly higher in cases with size 2 suture than in those with size 1 suture (86.9% vs. 93.5%, $p = 0.033$).

Q11. What are the Future fertility risks?

Draft recommendations: No significant adverse obstetrical outcome in women who received a uterine compression suture compared with those who did not receive a suture for PPH management.

The rate of subsequent pregnancies ranged from 11% to 75%, with an average of 32% (18 out of 57). However, no study had a follow-up period sufficient to assess long-term fertility. Additionally, many women who underwent compression sutures and faced a life-threatening delivery might be less inclined to pursue future pregnancies, complicating the analysis.

EMERGENCY PERIPARTUM HYSTERECTOMY

Background

Even 10 years ago, **Emergency Peripartum Hysterectomy** (EPH) was regarded as the **ultimate method of controlling Refractory PPH**. Today, with the advent of many non-surgical measures and conservative surgeries, coupled with the desire by the patients to preserve the uterus, it has become the desperate and terminal method of controlling refractory PPH. But having said that, the value of Obstetric hysterectomy has not gone down a bit also because in many hands and across many places in this vast country, it is often taken up quite early in PPH protocol as a life saving measure. It is a marker of SAMM and Near Miss also.

1. What is the preferred type of hysterectomy in PAS?
2. Any alternative to hysterectomy which is equally if not more useful?

Q12. What is the current epidemiology and prevalence rate of EPH?

Draft recommendations: This recommendation is based on Systemic Review and Meta-analysis only.

Incidence of EPH varies from 1 in 331 to 1 in 6978 deliveries worldwide. 1 in approx. 2000 in developed nations. In developing country like ours the incidence ranges from 1 in 400 to 1 in 2000. MMR ranges from 0 to 30% in EPH

Discussion: A 5 year systematic review and meta-analysis published in Obstet Gynecol. 2016 showed that hysterectomy complicated almost 1 per

1,000 deliveries.. One hundred twenty-eight studies were selected, including 7,858 women who underwent emergency peripartum hysterectomy, of whom 87% were multiparous. Hysterectomy complicated almost 1 per 1,000 deliveries (range 0.2-10.1). This prevalence is different among poorer (low and lower middle income) and richer (upper middle and high income) settings: 2.8 compared with 0.7 per 1,000 deliveries, respectively (relative risk 4.2, 95% confidence interval [CI] 4.0-4.5.

In a diverse country like India, the prevalence of hysterectomy has been reported as between 1.7 to 9.8 per 1000 within different regions of the country. PGI Chandigarh reported a prevalence of 6.9 per 1000 between 2014-15. A 2-year study at LLRM. Medical College, **Meerut**, between March 2021 to February 2023 showed 46 EOH were performed out of 7743 deliveries making an incidence of 5.04 per 1000 deliveries approx.

Q13. What are the absolute indications for EPH in today's obstetric practice?

Draft recommendations:

Common indications for EPH are:

- *Hemorrhage associated with:*
  - Uterine Atony unresponsive to oxytocics and conservative surgery
  - Placenta previa with or without morbid adhesion
  - Abruptio placentae
  - Uterine rupture with or without uterine trauma
  - External: Assault, fall or RTA.
- *Sepsis:* Clostridial infection, endomyometritis. not common now a days.

Discussion with Evidence

The 2016 meta-analysis showed that **most common indications were placental pathology (38%), uterine atony (27%), and uterine rupture (26%). A (previous) cesarean delivery is associated with a higher risk of emergency peripartum hysterectomy.**

In the 2023 meta-analysis in Obstet Gynaecol, the most common indications were placental pathology (38.0%, 95% CI 33.9-42.4), uterine atony (27.0%, 95% CI 24.6-29.5), and uterine rupture (21.2%, 95% CI 17.8-25.0). In lower middle-income countries, uterine rupture (44.5%, 95% CI 36.6-52.7) was the most common indication; placental pathology (48.4%, 95% CI 43.5-53.4) was most frequent in high-income settings. In the Meerut study published in 2023, the majority, 43.5% cases belonged to placenta accreta spectrum (PAS), followed by ruptured uterus (30.5%) and atonic postpartum hemorrhage (PPH) (26%).

Q14. What is the recommended technique for obstetric hysterectomy?

Draft recommendations

Preferred type of hysterectomy:

a. In most cases of obstetric hemorrhage, including EPH for rupture uterus, a quick **supracervical (also called subtotal)** hysterectomy is usually enough. It is quick, and effective in restoring near normal hemodynamic status in such cases.
b. In cases of PAS, **classical cesarean hysterectomy**—a thoroughly planned procedure after taking proper informed consent is recommended with placenta in situ.

Draft recommendation—technique: These days in most of the cases we go for this technique called **clamp, cut and drop technique.** In this technique, clamps are placed as usual, up to the uterine vessels, but they are not replaced by ligatures immediately, in order to save time. The clamps are replaced in the end by no. 1 Vicryl sutures, following double tie technique.

Care must be taken not to place lateral or downward traction on these clamps, which might tear friable tissues and cause bleeding that cannot be easily controlled. These clamps should be supported and not manipulated.

The vaginal cuff is secured by angle sutures which also includes the lower cardinal ligament pedicles, and the uterosacral pedicles. The surgeon may now choose to close the vaginal cuff with continuous or interrupted sutures. You may opt to leave the cuff open and to secure hemostasis of the anterior and posterior cuff edges with a continuous nonlocking suture.

The most important intra-operative problem is brisk hemorrhage and organ damage. Thus, simultaneous resuscitation with IV Fluids, blood and components should be continued to maintain adequate perfusion of the organs.

Q15. Any alternative to hysterectomy which is equally if not more useful?

Alternatives to hysterectomy:

A. A very recent publication in the J Endovasc Ther, May 2024 showed that meta-analysis comparing the effectiveness of uterine artery embolization (UAE) versus peripartum hysterectomy for acute refractory PPH control. The UAE population required less PRBC transfusion (MD: -7.39; 95% CI: -14.73 to -0.04; $p = 0.05$) and had shorter hospital stay (MD: -3.22; 95% CI: -5.42 to -1.02; $p = 0.004$). Although Lower mortality rates were noted for UAE in the pooled data, but it was not statistically significant. UAE also showed lower procedural complications (16.45% vs. 28.8%), meaning less ureter and bladder injuries (OR: 0.05; 95% CI: 0.01-0.38; $p = 0.004$ and OR: 0.02; 95% CI: 0.00-0.15; $p<0.001$, respectively). Only 35 (6%) required conversion to hysterectomy, while 27 (4.6%) underwent re-embolization with 100% bleeding control. UAE also did not hinder fertility, with normal menstruation restored in 19 patient.

B. *Conservative surgical treatment in PAS:* BMC Pregnancy childbirth Systematic Review and meta-analysis in July 2024 (this month) observed that cesarean hysterectomy as a traditional therapeutic intervention for placenta accreta spectrum (PAS) has been associated with serious morbidity, conservative management has been used in many institutions to treat women with PAS. This systematic review aims to compare maternal outcomes according to conservative management or cesarean hysterectomy in women with placenta accreta spectrum disorders.

   Results: Eight studies were included in the meta-analysis. Compared with cesarean hysterectomy, PAS women undergoing conservative management showed lower estimated blood loss [WMD - 1623.83; 95% CI: -2337.87, -909.79], required fewer units of packed red blood cells [WMD - 2.37; 95% CI: -3.70, -1.04] and units of fresh frozen plasma transfused [WMD - 0.40; 95% CI: -0.62, -0.19], needed a shorter mean operating time [WMD - 73.69; 95% CI: -90.52, -56.86], and presented decreased risks of bladder injury [RR 0.24; 95% CI: 0.11, 0.50], ICU admission [RR 0.24; 95% CI: 0.11, 0.52] and coagulopathy [RR 0.20; 95% CI: 0.06, 0.74], but increased risk for endometritis [RR 10.91; 95% CI: 1.36, 87.59] and readmission [RR 8.99; 95% CI: 4.00, 12.21]. The incidence of primary or delayed hysterectomy rate was 25% (95% CI: 19-32, I^2 = 40.88%) and the use of uterine arterial embolization rate was 78% (95% CI: 65-87, I^2 = 48.79%) in conservative management. This meta-analysis concluded that Conservative management could be an effective alternative to cesarean hysterectomy when women with PAS desire to preserve the uterus and are informed about the limitations of conservative management.

BIBLIOGRAPHY

1. Burchell RC. Physiology of internal iliac artery ligation. J Obstet Gynaecol Br Commonw. 1968;75:642–651.
2. Escobar M, Nassar AH, Theron G, et al. FIGO recommendations on the management of postpartum hemorrhage 2022. Int J Gynaecol Obstet. 2022;157 (Suppl 1): 3-50.
3. Joshi VM, Otiv SR, Majumder R, et al. Internal iliac artery ligation for arresting postpartum hemorrhage. BJOG. 2007;114:356-61.
4. Ledee N, Ville Y, Musset D, et al. Management in intractable obstetric haemorrhage: an audit study on 61 cases. Eur J Obstet Gynecol Reprod Biol. 2001;94:189-96.
5. Morel O, Malartic CJ, Muhlstein JE, et al. Pelvic arterial ligations for severe post-partum hemorrhage. Indications and techniques. J Visc Surg. 2011;148: 95-102.
6. Osanan GC, Charry RC, Alves ALL. (2021). Non-conservative and Conservative Surgical Management of PPH. [online] Available from https://www.glowm.

com/article/heading/vol-13--obstetric-emergencies--nonconservative-and-conservative-surgical-management-of-pph/id/413063 [Last accessed November, 2025].

7. Papp Z, Tóth-Pál E, Papp C, et al. Hypogastric artery ligation for intractable pelvic hemorrhage. Int J Gynecol Obstet. 2006;92(1):27-31.
8. Selçuk İ, Uzuner B, Boduç E, et al. Step-by-step ligation of the internal iliac artery. J Turk Ger Gynecol Assoc. 2019;20(2):123-128.
9. Sentilhes L, Trichot C, Resch B, et al. Fertility and pregnancy outcomes following uterine devascularization for severe postpartum haemorrhage. Hum Reprod. 2008;23:1087-92.
10. Unal O, Kars B, Buyukbayrak EE, et al. The effectiveness of bilateral hypogastric artery ligation for obstetric hemorrhage in three different underlying conditions and its impact on future fertility. J Matern Fetal Neonatal Med. 2011;24:1273-6.

CHAPTER 10

Traumatic Postpartum Hemorrhage

Rajesh Sharma, Sushil Chawla

Q1. What are the common causes of PPH? How Atonic PPH is differentiated from other causes of PPH?

Draft recommendations: To confirm that lacerations are a source of bleeding, careful inspection of the vagina, cervix, and uterus is essential. Sometimes bleeding may be caused by both atony and trauma, especially after forceps or vacuum-assisted vaginal delivery.

Evidence: When evaluating a patient who is bleeding, it may be helpful to consider "the 4 Ts" mnemonic device- tone, trauma, tissue and thrombin. Abnormal uterine tone is estimated to cause 70–80% of postpartum hemorrhage and usually should be suspected first as the etiology of postpartum hemorrhage.

Initial evaluation attempts to differentiate uterine atony from genital tract lacerations. Atony is identified by a boggy, soft uterus during bimanual examination and by expression of clots and hemorrhage during uterine massage. Persistent bleeding despite a firm, well-contracted uterus suggests that hemorrhage most likely is from lacerations. Bright red blood further suggests arterial bleeding. To confirm that lacerations are a source of bleeding, careful inspection of the vagina, cervix, and uterus is essential. Sometimes bleeding may be caused by both atony and trauma, especially after instrumental delivery.

Q2. What is uterine rupture? What is uterine dehiscence?

Draft Recommendations: Uterine rupture is a catastrophic condition requiring the notice of the obstetric history, antepartum and intrapartum factors to know the cause and manage it appropriately.

Evidence: A uterine rupture is a complete division of all three layers of the uterus: the endometrium (inner epithelial layer), myometrium (smooth muscle layer), and perimetrium (serosal outer surface).

Uterine dehiscence is a similar condition characterized by incomplete division of the uterus that does not penetrate all layers. Uterine dehiscence can produce a uterine window—a thinning of the uterine wall that may allow the fetus to be seen through the myometrium. Often uterine dehiscence is an occult finding in an asymptomatic patient.

Q3. What is the incidence of uterine rupture in scarred and unscarred uterus? What is the effect of uterine rupture on maternal and neonatal mortality?

Draft recommendations: The rate of uterine rupture is approximately 1% for women with one previous cesarean delivery versus 3.9% for those with greater than one previous cesarean delivery. Overall, it is estimated that one uterine rupture occurs for every 5,000 to 7,000 births.

Maternal mortality rates associated with rupture of scarred uterus is 0.1% whereas it is 10% with the rupture of unscarred uterus. The neonatal mortality rate with ruptured scarred uterus and unscarred uterus is 6% and 25% respectively.

Evidence: With quick surgical intervention and resuscitation, most women survive a uterine rupture. Although rare in an unscarred uterus, clinically significant uterine rupture occurs in 0.6 to 0.7 percent of vaginal births after cesarean delivery in women with a low transverse or unknown uterine scar. The risk increases significantly with previous classical incisions or uterine surgeries, and to a lesser extent with shorter intervals between pregnancies or a history of multiple cesarean deliveries, particularly in women with no previous vaginal deliveries.

Q4. What are the risk factors associated with Uterine Inversion and the appropriate management?

Draft recommendations: Uterine inversion refers to the collapse of the fundus into the uterine cavity. It carries a high risk of mortality due to hemorrhage and shock. The incidence is from 1 in 2000 to 1 in 20,000 vaginal deliveries.

Evidence: The risk factors associated with uterine inversion include alone or in combination include:

- Fundal placental implantation
- Uterine atony
- Cord traction applied before placental separation.
- Abnormally adhered placentation such as with the accrete syndromes.

Uterus should be replaced quickly. Placenta is usually attached, and it should not be removed. The replacement of uterus to its normal position is done by manual method. If manual method fails, it should be attempted again under tocolytic cover. If manual replacement of uterus fails even under tocolysis, laparotomy and surgical methods of uterine replacement may be required.

Q5. What is the incidence and risk factors of perineal hematomas?

Draft recommendations: Puerperal perineal hematoma is seen in 1 in 300 deliveries.

Labial, rectal, pelvic pressure or pain, or vital sign deterioration may be the only symptom of genital tract hematomas and may not be recognized until hours after delivery.

Evidence:: A potential space exists adjacent to the vaginal wall mucosa, extending from the vulva inferiorly to the extraperitoneal space superiorly, bounded by the broad ligament and other peritoneal reflections onto the bladder, uterus and rectum. As it is contiguous with the paravesical, parametrial and pararectal spaces, hemorrhage in one connective tissue space readily spreads to other. The vaginal venous plexus intercommunicates with the inferior and middle hemorrhoidal veins as well as with the inferior vesical plexus, and this entire venous pool becomes tremendously engorged during in third trimester of pregnancy. The levator ani muscles divide the paravaginal space into an supralevator fossa and infralevator fossa.

Paravaginal hematoma is an unavoidable obstetrical complication, usually due to the traction and rupture of paravaginal veins by the oncoming presenting part. Puerperal hematomas occur in 1:300 to 1:1500 deliveries.

The risk factors for development of puerperal hematomas are nulliparity, infant over 4000 grams, severe preeclampsia, prolonged second stage of labor, operative vaginal delivery, multifetal pregnancy, vulvar varicosities, or clotting disorders.

A paravaginal hematoma is typically confined to the lower compartment; however, it may extend superiorly into the supralevator and extraperitoneal space. Surgical evacuation may be complicated by the difficulty in accessing this space.

Labial, rectal, pelvic pressure or pain, swelling, ecchymosis or vital sign deterioration and urinary retention may be the only symptoms of infralevator genital tract hematomas, while supralevator hematomas give no external manifestations and may not be recognized until hours after delivery. Early diagnosis could be made more often by digital examination of the pelvis after the third stage of labor.

CT scan imaging is used to assess the spread and extension of hematoma. (especially the supralevator) Treatment varies depending upon site, size, spread of hematoma, hemodynamic status of patient and surgical preferences.

Once identified most genital tract hematomas can be managed conservatively. However rapid progressive enlargement of hematoma. Particularly in the setting of abnormal vital signs, indicate a need for incision and drainage. One reason that opening of hematomas is reserved is that often a single bleeding source is not identified when hematoma is incised. Exploration with suturing or packing is needed to achieve hemostasis.

Arterial embolization is another option for management of a hematoma and should be considered as a possibility before opening the hematoma.

Supralevator hematomas require laparotomy and internal iliac artery ligation.

Q6. What is colporrhexis?

Draft recommendations: Colporrhexis is an uncommon complication, which is often missed and causes significant morbidity and mortality.

Colporrhexis is defined as rupture of vaginal vault or upper one third of the vaginal wall, and was first coined in 1875 by Hugenberger, it occurs spontaneously or due to trauma as told by Resnick L. Primary colporrhexis has been described as a vaginal vault tear not associated with cervical or uterine extension while secondary colporrhexis is a vaginal vault tear which is associated with a rupture that has originated in the uterus or cervix and then extended to involve the vagina. Incomplete colporrhexis include rupture of vaginal epithelium and the muscularis, whereas complete includes overlying peritoneum as well in a study by Sahu.

As per Sharma KK most cases are of traumatic origin associated with unskilled instrumental delivery, vaginal birth after C-section, myomectomy, precipitate labor and injudicious use of oxytocics especially misoprostol in labor. A misdirection of the uterine axis due to a pendulous abdomen leading to marked anteversion of the uterus, ventroflexion of the uterus and prolapse leading to altered blood supply to the vagina are the other factors responsible.

Diagnosis of colporrhexis is clinical. Ultrasound abdomen and pelvis are required to assess associated intraperitoneal hemorrhage. Management depends on the maternal hemodynamics and extent of tear. In a stable patient without excessive hemorrhage or evidence of retroperitoneal hematoma, suturing of the laceration can be done by vaginal route under anesthesia. If patient is hemodynamically unstable with signs of inaccessible extension or retroperitoneal hematoma laparotomy and appropriate management is mandatory.

BIBLIOGRAPHY

1. American College of Obstetricians and Gynecologists. Clinical management guidelines for obstetrician-gynecologists: postpartum hemorrhage. ACOG Practice Bulletin No. 183. Obstet Gynecol. 2017;130(4):e168-86.
2. Baskett TF. Acute uterine inversion: a review of 40 cases. J Obstet Gynaecol Can. 2002;24:953-6.
3. Committee on Practice Bulletins-Obstetrics. Practice Bulletin No. 198 Summary: Prevention and Management of Obstetric Lacerations at Vaginal Delivery. Obstet Gynecol. 2018;132(3):795-7.
4. Cunningham FG, Leveno KJ, Bloom SL, et al. Williams Obstetrics, 26th edition. USA: McGraw Hill/Medical; 2022.
5. Lalonde A; International Federation of Gynecology and Obstetrics. Prevention and treatment of postpartum haemorrhage in low-resource settings. International J Gynecol Obstet. 2012;117:108-18.

6. Ozdemir I, Yucel N, Yucel O. Rupture of the pregnant uterus: A 9-year review. Arch Gynecol Obstet, 2005;272(3):229-31.
7. Rafi J, Muppala H. Retroperitoneal haematomas in obstetrics: literature review. Arch Gynecol Obstet. 2010;281:435-41.
8. Resnick L, Muller HW. Colporrhexis with a report of a case of spontaneous primary rupture of the posterior vaginal vault during labour. South African Med J. 1995;27(8):818-21.
9. Sahu L. A 10year analysis of uterine rupture in a teaching institution. J Obstet Gynaecol India, 2006;56(5):502-6.
10. Saleem Z, Rydhström H. Vaginal haematoma during parturition: a population-based study. Acta Obstet Gynecol Scand. 2004;83(6):560.
11. Sharma KK, Firth KM. Primary complete colporrhexis in primigravida. Br J Obstet Gynaecol. 1993;100(12):1142-4.
12. Tahseen S, Griffiths M. Vaginal birth after two caesarean sections (VBAC-2)-a systematic review with meta-analysis of success rate and adverse outcomes of VBAC-2 versus VBAC-1 and repeat (third) caesarean sections. BJOG. 2010; 117(1):5-19.
13. Zahn CM, Yeomans ER. Postpartum haemorrhage: placenta accreta, uterine inversion, and puerperal haematomas. Clin Obstet Gynecol, 1990;33:422-31.

CHAPTER 11

Secondary Postpartum Hemorrhage

Sushil Chawla

Q1. What constitutes "secondary postpartum hemorrhage"? What is the approximate load of the secondary PPH on the health system?

Draft recommendations:

- Secondary PPH is defined as any significant vaginal bleeding that occurs between 24 hours after placental delivery and during the following 6 weeks
- Secondary postpartum hemorrhage (SPPH) is an important complication postnatally which requires quick response from an obstetrician. The pressure of secondary PPH on the healthcare system is often underestimated.

Evidence

Definition: The definition of the secondary PPH is not clear, unlike the definition of primary PPH, there is no clear or standard definition for quantity of the blood loss associated with secondary PPH, and clinical expressions of this definition vary from 'increased lochia' to massive bleeding. The diagnosis is therefore all too often subjective, which may account for the numerous variations in reported incidence. *The international consensus has come to limit the later period to six weeks.*

Load on health care system: Secondary PPH or late PPH has been troubling the obstetrician and putting load on the health resources, however when you put the term in Google search engine or pubmed or even Cochrane database the number of studies, metanalysis, systematic reviews are very none to very few, thus putting the red light in the mind of all about this life-threatening and potentially fatal condition.

Primary postpartum hemorrhage (PPH) has been extensively studied; however, in comparison there is limited literature on SPPH as the number of women affected by SPPH is relatively small compared to the number of women affected by primary postpartum hemorrhage however it can cause serious complications if the recognition of this condition is delayed. The incidence of SPPH has been reported to be 0.2–2%. It is one of the most common indications for readmission after delivery and the incidence is highest in second week after delivery followed by third week. One study reported that as many as 22% of patients with SPPH required admission to the intensive care unit. As SPPH usually occurs in the second week after delivery, the time at which most patients are discharged from the hospital may contribute to the delay in its detection.

Research gaps: A need for clear cut definition will help in estimating the load on the healthcare system. This has to be done by robust collection of data in the retrospective studies and planning a system for the SPPH or secondary hemorrhage after an abortion.

Q2. What are the risk factors and causes of secondary postpartum hemorrhage?

Draft recommendations:

- SPPH is a relatively unexplored issue and there is limited evidence, regarding risk factors and it is important to identify the predictive factors for secondary PPH.
- Etiology of secondary PPH is diverse.

Evidence

Risk factors for SPPH: A Cochrane review in 2002 did not identify any randomized controlled trials that sufficiently informed the management SPPH. Since this review, there have been several studies outlining management options; however, in comparison limited studies have attempted to explore the risk factors, with only three key recent studies on this topic. Debost Legrand, et al., Marchant et al., and Hoveyda and MacKenzie identified Primary PPH, maternal age >35 years. history of SPPH, prolonged or incomplete third stage, maternal smoking, incomplete third stage, third trimester hospital admission, vaginal bleeding prior to 24 weeks gestation and manual removal of placenta to be associated with SPPH. While primary PPH appears consistently as a risk factor, other findings are less conclusive. Antenatal use of anticoagulation, High BMI, GDM are few of the other risk or predictive factors for SPPH.

Causes of SPPH: The most common causes of secondary PPH are retained products of conception (RPOC), Placental site subinvolution (delayed closure of the vessels at the placental attachment site), abnormally invasive placentation, postpartum endometritis with or without scar dehiscence and coagulopathies. Other causes include uterine arteriovenous fistulas (AVFs), uterine artery pseudoaneurysms, uterine rupture with vessel injury, choriocarcinoma, cervical carcinoma, among others.

Research gaps: Further research is warranted with the aim to identify risk factors and causative factors for SPPH to inform clinical management and decrease maternal morbidity.

Q3. What is the role of USS and color Doppler in diagnosis and treatment of secondary PPH?

Draft recommendations:

- Ultrasonography with color Doppler flow imaging is the cornerstone and holds the key in the diagnosis of secondary PPH.
- MRI and interventional radiology acts as an adjunct to ultrasound for diagnosis and treatment of secondary PPH.

Evidence: Pelvic ultrasonography and doppler studies can be performed via a transabdominal or transvaginal approach. The normal postpartum uterus has a variable sonographic appearance from containing anechoic fluid or echogenic material. Thus, the clinical context is essential for interpreting the significance of these findings.

Retained Products of conception (RPOC): It means residual fetal, placental, or other decidual tissue remaining within the uterus after delivery. On grayscale USS, RPOC may appear as a hyperechoic or mixed-echogenicity mass(>10 mm) in the endometrial cavity, a heterogeneously thickened endometrial stripe, an irregular interface of endo-myometrial junction. The presence of vascularity in a thickened Endometrium or endometrial mass is highly suggestive of RPOC and degree of vascularity can be divided into four groups by comparing endometrial vascularity to the adjacent normal myometrial vascularity. Since RPOC may be avascular, the absence of color Doppler flow does not exclude the diagnosis. Evaluation with MRI typically shows an endometrial polypoid mass with heterogeneous signals on T1- and T2-weighted images. Variable enhancement can be seen on postcontrast images based on the vascularity of the RPOC.

Endometritis: Endometritis is a clinical diagnosis, and the infected endometrium can demonstrate normal postpartum sonographic features without any specific imaging findings of infection or it may appear as - fluid and echogenic debris within the endometrial cavity, thickened endometrium and heterogeneous appearance with increased vascularity or the ring-down artefact. However, endometrial gas can be a normal finding for up to 3 weeks after delivery in up to 20% of healthy postpartum patients.

Subinvolution of placental site: US may show hypoechoic tortuous vessels within the myometrium at the location of the prior placental implantation site. Color Doppler US manifests prominent vascular flow with increased PSV and a low resistance waveform. There are no reports describing the CT and MRI features of subinvolution. Angiographically, subinvolution presents as hypertrophied uterine arteries. The uterine parenchyma rapidly opacifies and drains into large pelvic veins but no direct communication between the artery and vein is visualized.

Uterine arteriovenous malformation: The UAVMs occur when there is a direct communication between the arterial and venous systems without an intervening capillary bed. US findings are often variable and non-specific, including myometrial heterogeneity or thickening. Sometimes an ill-defined heterogeneous intramural or endometrial mass may be seen, containing multiple cystic or tubular structures. Color Doppler shows multidirectional flow with aliasing and a mosaic pattern associated with turbulent high-velocity flow. Timmerman et al. reported that the peak systolic velocity (PSV) appears to be useful for predicting low- and high-risk patients with uterine AVM. The MRI findings of true AVM include a bulky uterus, a focal mass with disruption of the junctional zone, multiple serpiginous flow voids within the lesion, and prominent parametrial vessels. Angiography is the gold standard for diagnosing AVM: findings include a dilated, tortuous uterine artery feeding a hyper vascular uterine mass and early venous return to an enlarged vein.

Uterine artery pseudoaneurysm: Pseudoaneurysms usually result from laceration or injury of the arterial wall and are often associated with surgical procedures such as operative delivery and D&C. The location of a pseudoaneurysm after vaginal delivery may include the vaginal artery or obturator artery, while pseudoaneurysm after cesarean delivery usually involves the uterine artery. The US findings of uterine artery pseudoaneurysm should show bidirectional swirling arterial flow, which may resemble the yin-yang symbol (yin-yang sign). During spectral analysis, a "to-and-fro" waveform should be seen at the neck of the pseudoaneurysm, and blood passes into and out of the pseudoaneurysm. Pseudoaneurysm may appear as a flow void on T2-weighted MRI with intense enhancement on gadolinium-enhanced MRI, and often surrounded by a hyperintense hematoma on T1-weighted imaging. However, MRI is not an ideal modality for emergency use. Angiography can clearly demonstrate and confirm the presence of a pseudoaneurysm, and facilitates subsequent embolization.

Gestational trophoblastic disease: The US findings of invasive mole and choriocarcinoma are heterogeneous, echogenic, hypervascular uterine masses with possible myometrial invasion. Areas of necrosis and hemorrhage can be seen within choriocarcinoma. The hyper vascular nature of these tumors can be helpful in detecting myometrial invasion, although invasion is not always detectable. Choriocarcinoma is usually seen as an intrauterine mass with heterogeneous high signal intensity on T2-weighted imaging and marked peripheral enhancement with central necrosis on postcontrast images. Enhancing parametrial soft tissue is characteristic of local spread. Metastatic disease is also detected by MRI, particularly within the pelvic organs and lymph nodes. The imaging findings of GTD may overlap with those of RPOC.

Q4. What are the different treatment modalities in the specific treatment of secondary PPH? What is the role of Interventional radiology, hysteroscopy in treatment of secondary PPH?

Draft recommendations:

- Resuscitation forms an important step in the management of secondary PPH
- The different options for managing the case of secondary PPH includes - medical(Antibiotics, uterotonics, antifibrinolytics), surgical management (uterus conserving and hysterectomy), interventional radiological management.

Resuscitation: 95% of women with secondary PPH present within the first month after delivery. The amount of blood loss at presentation varies but most patients are hemodynamically stable. Approximately 10% of cases present with massive hemorrhage. Restoration of circulating blood volume should be achieved by gaining intravenous access with two large-bore cannulae and administering intravenous fluids initially with physiological saline and then with plasma expanders until blood is available. High concentration oxygen (10–15 l/min) should be administered by a tight-fitting mask. Close observation of vital signs including pulse, blood pressure, oxygen saturation and urine output should be maintained throughout resuscitation. Blood and blood products should be given according to blood loss, rather than waiting and using the response to initial fluid administration and hemoglobin and coagulation results as the trigger for the infusion of blood. Identification of the cause of bleeding should then be made and further management planned accordingly.

Clinical signs and symptoms at the time of presentation may include offensive lochia, abdominal cramping, uterine tenderness, pyrexia, enlarged uterus and an open cervical os.

Baseline blood tests should include full blood count, coagulation studies, C-reactive protein and serum hCG. Vaginal swabs should be taken at the time of examination for aerobic as well as anaerobic bacterial growth, including swabs from episiotomy or vaginal tear sites. In women with signs of infection, a mid-stream urine specimen should be collected and, if there is fever, blood cultures should be obtained.

Medical: Antibiotics—endometritis is likely to play a significant role in many cases of secondary PPH, and the majority of women are prescribed antibiotics. In a 3-year study of almost 20,000 women, 132 women (0.69%) had a secondary PPH, and 97% of these were treated with antibiotics 2. However, only 75% of these women had microbiological specimens collected; of these, a positive culture was obtained in only 13.5%. Although infection may not be confirmed in a large population of cases, we recommend that antibiotics are always given for secondary PPH.

Uterotonics—oxytocin, methylergometrine, carboprost or misoprostol can be used to cause the contraction of the uterus. The bolus dose of the injection oxytocin can be followed by infusion.

Tranexamic acid—The drug can be used in an injectable form or the oral preparation and continued for a variable period of 24-72 hrs.

Hormonal therapy—the hormones used in this condition are COC's, GnRH analogs there are no data available about the efficacy of hormones in this condition.

Surgical: Uterine evacuation—this forms the mainstay of treatment in cases of RPOC. The procedure may be carried out under USS guidance as the uterus is soft and there are high chances of uterine perforation.

Uterine balloon tamponade—this is carried out to buy time in an emergency and may act as a definite treatment in a few cases.

Hysteroscopy and resection—this procedure is an ideal one for the removal of the RPOC using a resectoscope with the energy source.

Hysterectomy—this is generally done as the last procedure, when the other treatments have failed or the patient is hemodynamically compromised, necessitating this radical surgery.

Interventional radiological management: This is actually undertaken as a package for the diagnosis and treatment in the same sitting after a USS has indicated the presence of pseudoaneurysm or UAVM. Uterine artery embolization is regarded as the gold standard of treatment for pseudoaneurysms. As the uterus is preserved, and the risk of complications due to hysterectomy was avoided. The prohibitive cost of setting up the center has limited its use only at the tertiary care centers.

BIBLIOGRAPHY

1. Alexander J, Thomas PW, Sanghera J. (2002). Treatments for secondary postpartum haemorrhage. Cochrane Database Syst Rev. 2002;(1):CD002867.
2. Fox R, Aitken G, Mooney SS. Management of secondary postpartum haemorrhage: A systematic review. Eur J Obstet Gynecol Reprod Biol. 2023; 282:116-23.
3. Fox R, Anderson J, Young N, et al. Medical management of secondary postpartum haemorrhage: A prospective cohort study. Aust N Z J Obstet Gynaecol. 2023; 63:52-8.
4. Groom KM, Jacobson TZ. The management of secondary postpartum hemorrhage. In: B-Lynch C, Keith LG, Lalonde AB, Karoshi M (Eds). Textbook of postpartum haemorrhage. A comprehensive guide to evaluation, management and surgical intervention (pp. 316-324). Duncow: Sapiens Publishing; 2006.

5. Hamel CC, van Wessel S, Carnegy A, et al. Diagnostic criteria for retained products of conception—A scoping review. Acta Obstet Gynecol Scand. 2021;100: 2135-3.
6. Hoveyda F, MacKenzie IZ. Secondary postpartum haemorrhage: incidence, morbidity and current management. BJOG. 2001;108:927-30.
7. Iraha Y, Okada M, Toguchi M, et al. Multimodality imaging in secondary postpartum or postabortion hemorrhage: retained products of conception and related conditions. Jpn J Radiol. 2018;36:12-22.
8. Kothari A, Hay K, Rudra T. Risk Factors for Secondary Postpartum Haemorrhage: A Retrospective Study. J Med Res Surg. 2002;3(2):31-5.
9. Loya MF, Garcia-Reyes K, Gichoya J, et al. Uterine Artery Embolization for Secondary Postpartum Hemorrhage. Tech Vasc Interv Radiol. 2021;24(1): 100728.
10. Shinohara S, Okuda Y, Hirata S, Suzuki K. Predictive factors for secondary postpartum hemorrhage: a case-control study in Japan. J Matern Fetal Neonatal Med. 2002;35(20):3943-7.
11. Young N, Quinlivan J, Fox R, et al. Economic cost of secondary postpartum haemorrhage: A case-control study at a tertiary hospital in Australia. Aust N Z J Obstet Gynaecol. 2023;63:308-13.
12. Zubor P, Kajo K, Dokus K, et al. Recurrent secondary postpartum hemorrhages due to placental site vessel subinvolution and local uterine tissue coagulopathy. BMC Pregnancy Childbirth. 2014;14:80.

CHAPTER 12

Postpartum Hemorrhage and Special Situations

Madhva Prasad

Q1. What are the recommendations regarding PPH in multiple pregnancy?

Draft recommendations: A higher level of preparedness for postpartum hemorrhage (PPH) should be kept ready while managing multiple pregnancies. Management of PPH in twin pregnancies follow similar recommendations as management of standard guidelines. Among women with a multiple pregnancy and cesarean delivery, prophylactic tranexamic acid does not reduce the incidence of any blood loss-related outcomes.

Discussion/summary of evidence: Multiple pregnancy is a well-known risk factor PPH. Obstetricians must always be prepared for prevention and management of PPH in multiple pregnancy. The standard management of PPH should be instituted in multiple pregnancies. Though tranexamic acid has been advocated for prevention of PPH, it may not be effective in multiple pregnancies. A secondary of the TRAAP trial (involving more than 4500 mothers with twin pregnancies) suggested that there is there may be no specific benefits of adding prophylactic tranexamic acid for prevention of PPH among twin pregnancies undergoing cesarean section. (The occurrence of PPH was 42% in tranexamic acid group and 44% in placebo group (risk ratio of 0.97, *p* value 0.86).

Q2. What are the recommendations regarding PPH in severe preeclampsia?

Draft recommendations: A higher level of preparedness for PPH should be kept ready when managing patients with severe preeclampsia, especially when patient is on magnesium sulphate. Carbetocin is recommended (rather than oxytocin) in the prevention of postpartum hemorrhage in women with severe preeclampsia. When complicated by coagulopathy, early initiation of LMWH is recommended.

Discussion/summary of evidence: Postpartum hemorrhage is much higher among those with hypertensive disorders of pregnancy (relative risk of 1.11). Those with severe preeclampsia have a much higher risk of postpartum hemorrhage compared to those without severe features (relative risk of 1.52). Such risk of PPH is much higher among those who are on magnesium sulphate (relative risk of 1.93). This is probably explained by the tocolytic properties of magnesium sulphate. Management of PPH in preeclampsia follows the general principles of management of PPH. Methylergometrine is to be avoided where hypertensive disorder cannot be safely excluded. Though carbetocin and oxytocin may have equivalent benefit for prevention of PPH among patients with severe preeclampsia, carbetocin offers the significant advantage of lesser volume of fluid per dose, which is of importance in severe preeclampsia. Hence, carbetocin may be considered as a valid alternative compared to oxytocin. Disseminated intravascular coagulation is an established complication of severe preeclampsia, which can in turn lead to postpartum hemorrhage due to consumptive coagulopathy. Initiation of low molecular weight heparin is suggested after recovery from bleeding risk, and has the composite impact of reduction of coagulopathy-associated problems.

Q3. What are the recommendations regarding PPH in patients who were on medications for preventing preeclampsia (aspirin)?

Draft recommendations: Discontinue aspirin at least 7 days prior to anticipated delivery to prevent the risk of PPH. Earlier discontinuation may be considered in patients with obesity.

Discussion/summary of evidence: Usage of low-dose aspirin does not appear to increase the risk of PPH immaterial of maternal characteristics. Specifically, it does not increase the risk of postpartum hemorrhage if discontinued more than 7 days prior to the delivery. Patients with obesity may be at slightly higher risk than other patients.

Q4. What are the recommendations regarding PPH in patients with intrahepatic cholestasis of pregnancy?

Draft recommendations: No specific changes are recommended for management of PPH in patients with intrahepatic cholestasis of pregnancy

Discussion/summary of evidence: Very few studies have evaluated the intrahepatic cholestasis of pregnancy on postpartum blood loss. Overall there appears to be no major increase in PPH due to the condition.

Q5. What are the recommendations regarding PPH in patients with uterine fibroids?

Draft recommendations: Higher preparedness is needed for prevention and management of PPH when there is presence of fibroid, immaterial of mode of delivery and location of fibroid. PPH is higher with larger size of fibroid. Cesarean myomectomy increases the risk of intraoperative hemorrhage, blood transfusion and entails overall higher morbidity to the patient.

Discussion/summary of evidence: The frequency with which clinicians encounter fibroid uterus in pregnancy has increased over time. Postpartum hemorrhage is higher in the presence of uterine fibroid (odds ratio of 1.2). Frequency of occurrence of postpartum hemorrhage appears to be similar, immaterial of vaginal delivery or cesarean section. A larger size of fibroid leads to more risk and higher volume of postpartum hemorrhage. Though the occurrence of PPH is higher in some types of locations more than the others, the possibility should be kept in mind at all times. (intramural 8.6%, subserosal 5.6% and submucosal 4.7% respectively). Performance of planned Cesarean myomectomy has increased over the last many years. However, clinicians must be prepared to encounter intraoperative hemorrhage, and be prepared for prompt medical and surgical management of PPH when this is encountered.

Q6 What are the recommendations regarding PPH in patients who are obese?

Draft recommendations: Occurrence of PPH is higher among women with obesity. Women with obesity must be informed of the same and clinicians should be prepared for it. Women with obesity should be offered prevention of postpartum hemorrhage with single dose 100 mcg of intravenous carbetocin.

Discussion/summary of evidence: Polic et al. in their article "The Impact of Obesity on the Management and Outcomes of Postpartum Hemorrhage" note that women with obesity have higher amount of blood loss (p value 0.003), higher amount of uterotonic agents (p value 0.007), higher need for post-delivery/postoperative surgical interventions (p value 0.04), higher need for blood transfusion (p value 0.023) and higher amount of hemorrhage related morbidity (p value 0.02). El Behery et al. suggest that a single 100 µg IV carbetocin is more effective than IV oxytocin infusion for maintaining adequate uterine tone and preventing postpartum bleeding in obese nulliparous women undergoing emergency cesarean delivery.

BIBLIOGRAPHY

1. Cagino KA, Wiley RL, Ghose I, et al. Risk of Postpartum Haemorrhage in Hypertensive Disorders of Pregnancy: Stratified by Severity. Am J Perinatol. 2024;41(4), 396-402.
2. Chen J, Huai J, Lin L, et al. Low-dose aspirin in the prevention of pre-eclampsia in China: postpartum hemorrhage in subgroups of women according to their characteristics and potential bleeding risk. Chinese Med J (English). 2023;136(5):550-55.
3. El Behery MM, El Sayed G., El Hameed AA, et al. Carbetocin versus oxytocin for prevention of postpartum haemorrhage in obese nulliparous women undergoing emergency caesarean delivery. J Matern Fetal Neonat Med. 2016; 29(8):1257-60.
4. Escobar M, Nassar AH, Theron G, et al. FIGO recommendations on the management of postpartum hemorrhage 2022. Int J Gynaecol Obstet. 2022;157 (Suppl 1): 3-50.

5. Furrer R, Winter K, Schäffer L, et al. Postpartum Blood Loss in Women Treated for Intrahepatic Cholestasis of Pregnancy. Obstet Gynecol. 2016;128(5):1048-52.
6. Gong J, Chen Z, Zhang Y, et al. Risk-factor model for postpartum haemorrhage after caesarean delivery: a retrospective study based on 3498 patients. Sci Rep. 2022;12(1):22100.
7. Hagenbeck C, Hamza A, Kehl S, et al. Management of Intrahepatic Cholestasis of Pregnancy: Recommendations of the Working Group on Obstetrics and Prenatal Medicine-Section on Maternal Disorders. Geburtshilfe und Frauenheilkunde. 2021;81(8), 922-939.
8. Henderson JT, Vesco KK, Senger CA, et al. Aspirin Use to Prevent Preeclampsia and Related Morbidity and Mortality. Rockville: Agency for Healthcare Research and Quality (US). 2021
9. Huang Y, Ming X, Li Z. Feasibility and safety of performing caesarean myomectomy: a systematic review and meta-analysis. J Matern Fetal Neonat Med. 2022;35(13):2619-27.
10. Kilicci C, Ozkaya E, Karakus R, et al. Early low molecular weight heparin for postpartum hemorrhage in women with pre-eclampsia. Is it effective to prevent consumptive coagulopathy? J Matern Fetal Neonat Med. 2020;33(3): 410-4.
11. Lan Y, Xu A, Lu X, et al. Risk factors for postpartum hemorrhage in twin pregnancies with caesarean section. Front Med. 2024;10:1301807.
12. Li H, Hu Z, Fan Y, et al. The influence of uterine fibroids on adverse outcomes in pregnant women: a meta-analysis. BMC Pregnancy Childbirth. 2024; 24(1):345.
13. Pergialiotis V, Bellos I, Constantinou T, et al. Magnesium sulfate and risk of postpartum uterine atony and hemorrhage: A meta-analysis. European Journal of Obstet Gynecol Reprod Biol. 2021;256:158-64.
14. Polic A, Curry TL, Louis JM. The impact of obesity on the management and outcomes of postpartum haemorrhage. Am J Perinatol. 2022;39(6):652-7.
15. Reyes OA, Gonzalez GM. Carbetocin versus oxytocin for prevention of postpartum hemorrhage in patients with severe preeclampsia: a double-blind randomized controlled trial. J Obstet Gynaecol Can. 2011;33(11):1099-104.
16. Sentilhes L, Madar H, Le Lous M, et al. (2022). Tranexamic acid for the prevention of blood loss after caesarean among women with twins: a secondary analysis of the TRAnexamic Acid for Preventing Postpartum Haemorrhage Following a Caesarean Delivery randomized clinical trial. Am J Obstet Gynecol. 2022;227(6):889.e1-889.e17.
17. White KJ, Son M, Lundsberg LS, et al. Low-Dose Aspirin during Pregnancy and Postpartum Bleeding. Am J Perinatol. 2023;40(13):1390-7.
18. Zhao R, Wang X, Zou L, et al. Adverse obstetric outcomes in pregnant women with uterine fibroids in China: A multicenter survey involving 112,403 deliveries. PLOS One. 2017:12(11):e0187821.

13

CHAPTER

Tools and Resources

Saswati Sanyal Choudhury, Gowri Sayiprasad

TEACHING AND CASE AWARENESS: TEAM MEASURES FOR MANAGEMENT

Q1. Elaborate the teaching and evaluation aids that help in effective management of PPH resulting in upgradation of the skills of the health care provider.

- **Draft recommendations:** Teaching, detection and evaluation aids help in supporting the skills of the health worker. The health learning materials are visual, audio, audio-visual which can be used to teach and train workers.
- **Detection aids:** Graded under sheets, blood collection drape, calibrated drapes 300, 500 mL, MEOWS chart triggers are the available and recommended aids for postpartum hemorrhage (PPH) detection. No one method is superior over the other as mentioned in the FIGO practice recommendations 2022. Visual estimation of postpartum blood loss is frequently inaccurate. Objective methods of quantifying blood loss, which are superior to visual estimation, are more likely to detect PPH.
- **Treatment aids:** PPH trolleys or kits with contents on display with number of units, emergency resuscitation trolley or kits with contents and display of drugs, devices such as Bakri balloon, suction devices, anti-shock garment are the treatment aids available.
- **Teaching aids:** Charts in the antenatal area (pictures and local language), labor room and delivery area target different groups, i.e., patients/attenders and health care providers. Create the charts, apply the charts and strategies that are most easily understandable. Local language implementation for patient information charts. Training of the providers with visual, audio-visual aids have consistently reduced patient morbidity, especially in low resource settings. New obstetric care provider joining the team should be trained about audit of care and usage of drugs. Every society conference can be suggested to have a PPH drill involving select group of local midwives/staff/managers.
- **Evaluation aids:** Audit of near miss cases, stock availability, team response, random audit of data entry and staff simulation protocols in Special Situations should be performed routinely. The implementation of the recommendations should be monitored at the health-service level.

Interrupted time series, clinical audits or criterion-based clinical audits could be used to obtain relevant data related to the management of PPH.
Levels of prevention:

Primary prevention	• Importance of booking, triage ANC cards for high risk pregnancy • Blood checks • Supplements
Secondary prevention	• Training for identification and prompt action(medical/surgical) • Charts for drug usage and blood products
Tertiary prevention	• Early referral • Transport facilities

Q2. How can the protocols for skill development of health care personnel be implemented for their upgradation?

Draft recommendations: Strategies, care protocols, education programs need to be locally developed and stringently implemented for consistent skill development of health workers.

Birth preparedness and complication readiness (BP/CR) is a strategy to promote the timely use of skilled maternal and neonatal care, especially during childbirth, based on the theory that preparing for childbirth and being ready for complications reduces delays in obtaining this care.

Development of implementable strategies, local protocols upgradations and revision workshops, distance education programs are some of the regularly strategies.

Utilizing simulation and hands-on training for skill enhancement with repetition and practice of inter-disciplinary collaboration are areas that need definition.

Monitoring and evaluating PPH clinical guideline implementation: The implementation of the PPH clinical protocol should be monitored at all levels of care where maternity services are provided. Clinical audits or criterion-based audits can be used based on clearly defined review criteria and indicators, locally agreed. Constructive feedback from enhancers and mentors help in improving the performance of health care workers.

COMMUNICATION STRATEGIES

Q3.What are the standard communication pattern tools and how to incorporate them in a real time scenario?

Draft recommendations: Communication between members of the team and with the patient/attenders is crucial. Two of the most effective communication strategies clinicians use among themselves are the ISBARR and STICC.

Communication with the patient and her birthing partner is important, and clear information of what is happening should be given from the outset.

Communication between team members is the key to a good outcome. Clear and timely communication between surgical, anesthetic and hematology/blood transfusion services is one of the cornerstones to success. Define the roles and responsibilities of midwives, medical interns, medical officers, obstetric registrars, obstetricians, anesthetists and staff involved in the care of women with postpartum hemorrhage in both basic and comprehensive Emergency Obstetric Care (EmOC) health facilities.

Optimize within team coordination and teamwork enhancement is recommended.

Identify team members, hierarchy maintenance.

Define role of every member:

- *Team leader:* Clinically experienced, leads resuscitative and treatment strategy.
- *1-2 staff:* Clinical assistance, procedure, administer medication, documentation of events with timing.
- *1 staff:* Monitoring and clinical assistance, Counsels family/members accompanying patient.
- *1 manager/nonclinical member:* Helps for emergency transport; blood.

ISBARR: This is a regularly used method of communication in health care scenarios. (Introduction, Situation, Background, Assessment, Recommendations, Repeat back).

STICC: Situation, Task, Intent, Concern and Calibrate is the other strategy.

Establish effective, complete, clear, brief, timely and respectful communication between team members.

Team evaluation and appraisal post event (virtual and real time):

- Practice mock and random drills, empower staff to communicate with each other and mentors.
- *Audit real life situation:* reflect on individual and team performance improvement.
- Keep communications confidential.
- Lucid documentation.

Q4. Debriefing methods of all cases of PPH.

Draft recommendations: The main goal of debriefings has been to improve clinical outcomes by learning through discussion and reflection of events and then transferring that learning into clinical practice.

Regular timed meetings for appraisal after an event should have the key components of properly planned, honest reporting, confidentiality, learning and summary. Various debriefing tools and structures are in use, such as TALK (Target, Analysis, Learning, Key Actions), PEARLS (Promoting Excellence and Reflective Learning in Simulation) and REFLECT (Review the event, Encourage team participation, Focused feedback, Listen to each other, Emphasize key points, Communicate clearly, Transform the future).

The team leader or the key facilitator should lead the debriefing efforts after real time PPH scenarios.

Q5. How to establish communication within the community and enrich participation?

Draft recommendations: Frontline health workers such as ASHAs are the face of the health system within the rural community and would continue to remain the same in the future. They can be effectively used to enhance community participation.

Community awareness and participation

Community ↔ ASHA ↔ Health Center staff ↔ Hospital Staff ↔ Referral hospital.

These strategies attempt at improving the primary preventive methods of enhancing nutritional and health statuses of the mother, timely visits, recognizing danger signals, possibility of complications, referral facilities and transport. Effective and open-ended communication between community leaders and health care workers, doctors is bridged by the ASHA who are important keys in disbursing information. At the household level, ASHA/ANM sensitizes the key decision makers and pregnant women for right decision at right time and timely referral through preidentified transport for helping women access the services available as and when required. ASHA/ANM also promote and facilitate community involvement for collective action and shared responsibility through the community mobilization process. Through this process, community leaders and influential, non-governmental organizations, local government officials, health providers are encouraged to contribute to mobilization and establishment of community mechanisms for emergency funds and transportation.

SCOPE FOR RESEARCH

Q6. Can digital health applications be used for individual case management?

Draft recommendations: Better patient data management and increased healthcare access, especially in remote areas, have been made possible by the integration of digital platforms, electronic health records, telemedicine services, and mobile health apps.

In the current scenario, digital technology can be very effectively incorporated into the management of PPH scenario and in high-risk pregnancy management. ANCHAL (ANTENATAL NEONATAL and CHILD HEALTH SYSTEMS AND LOGISTICS TRACKING TOOL) are some of the tools developed by the government integrating community and other health workers. Telemedicine, telemonitoring and eHealth records can help in timely intervention as well as access to emergency care provider. Modules, training videos access can be made easy to access and redo.

Q7. How to bridge the gap between training and real-life situation management?

Draft recommendations: Simulation models need to be researched further to bridge the gap between reality and lab situations.

This is where the trainers and trainees can learn through virtual reality and simulators. These spaces provide learners with realistic learning experiences, build confidence and work awareness and prepare them for the challenges of real-world learning areas to perfect teamwork and communication skills.

The development of low and high-fidelity simulators and a guided training program for health workers can bridge this gap between theory and practical application of skills. This can be an area of further research. Clinical algorithms may be adopted, and AI based tools can be tested in resource poor settings.

BIBLIOGRAPHY

1. Kolbe M, Schmutz S, Seelandt JC, et al. Team debriefings in healthcare: aligning intention and impact. Br Med J. 2021;374:n2042.
2. Mavrides EAS, Chandraharan E, Collins P, et al. Prevention and management of post-partum haemorrhage: green-top guideline No 52. BJOG. 2017;124: e106-49.
3. Ministry of Health and Family Welfare Government of India Guidance Note on Prevention and Management of Postpartum Haemorrhage. Delhi: Ministry of Health and Family Welfare Government of India; 2015. pp. 7-9.
4. Mishra A, Singh AK, Parida SP, et al. Understanding Community Participation in Rural Health Care: A Participatory Learning and Action Approach. Front Public Health. 2022;10:860792.
5. Pali, J., Rajasuganya, & Logapriya. (2024). India's digital health odyssey: Foundations of Healthcare Technologies Society. A quarterly newsletter. [online] Available from https://fhts.ac.in/indias-digital-health-odyssey/ [Last accessed November, 2024].
6. Saleem M, Khan Collins TE, Akselrod S, et al. The promise of digital health technologies for integrated care for maternal and child health and non-communicable diseases. Br Med J. 2023;381:e071074.
7. Walker D, Fritz J, Olvera M, et al et al. PRONTO Low-Tech Obstetric Simulation and Team Training in Mexico Improves Patient Outcomes, and Evidence-Based Care at Birth. Obstet Gynecol. 2014;123(1):176S-7S.

8. WHO. WHO recommendations for the prevention and treatment of postpartum haemorrhage. Geneva: World Health Organization; 2012.
9. WHO. WHO recommendations on the assessment of postpartum blood loss and treatment bundles for postpartum haemorrhage. Geneva: World Health Organization; 2023.
10. World Health Organization. (2019). Definition of skilled health personnel providing care during childbirth: the 2018 joint statement by WHO, UNFPA, UNICEF, ICM, ICN, FIGO and IPA. [online] Available from https://www.who.int/publications/i/item/WHO-RHR-18.14 [Last accessed November, 2024].
11. World Health Organization. Recommendations on the assessment of postpartum blood loss and use of a treatment bundle for postpartum haemorrhage. Geneva: World Health Organization; 2023. pp. 26.

14

CHAPTER

Implementation and Training

Poonam Varma Shivkumar, Seema Mehrotra

The implementation of PPH–EEBR recommendation are to be considered by all stakeholders involved in the care of pregnant women at the international, national and local levels. There is a crucial need to increase access of women to health care and to strengthen the capacity at health-care facilities and providers of all levels to ensure they can provide high-quality services to all women giving birth. It is therefore vital that these recommendations be translated into care packages and programs at country and healthcare facility levels, where appropriate.

Q1. What would be preliminary preparations before commencing training on FOGSI PPH EEBR 2024?

Draft recommendations: Effective training to include development of pool of master trainers, identifying the training sites and optimum duration of training and developing training modules

Evidence summary: Foremost step in preparation of training will include identifying the core group from private and public facility. This core group will develop modules for master trainers using various standard guidelines. Master trainers will be specialist with minimum 5 yrs experience as teacher/trainer from Dept of OBS & GYN from different states who will be willing for the training.

Next step will be sensitization and training of master trainers for 7-10 days by core group regarding the way they will be conducting the training for the trainees using prespecified module which will include pretest assessment, theoretical lessons, skill practice, feedback loop and post test assessment. Another important component will include identifying the site of training and working out the logistics such as accommodation, food, teaching venue, modules printing, schedule of training, transport, preparing venue as per the sessions and teaching methodology, inviting master trainers and arranging their transport, accommodation, food and modules **(Flowchart 1)**.

Optimum duration of training will be 2 weeks for Medical officers and 3 weeks for technical staff. Training will be followed by final assessment and certification and posting the trained persons at appropriate facilities. This will be followed by mentoring visits at the trainees health facility by

Flowchart 1: Training cycle.

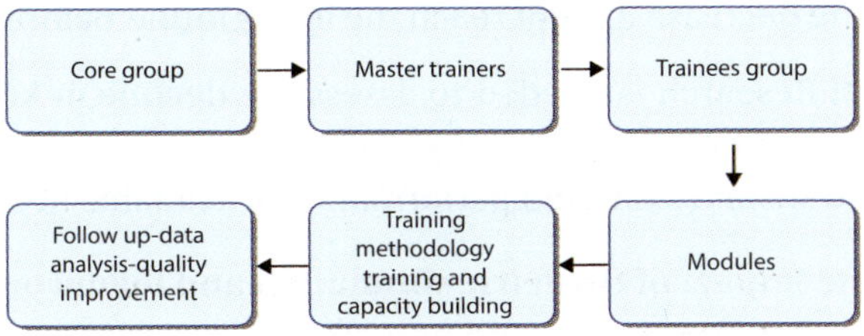

Master trainers, 3 times, 2 visits 3 monthly and last after 6 months and each visit outcome indicators and data to be evaluated and analyzed.

Research gap: What type of and how much training leads to optimum use of evidence based practices (EBPs) thereby improving patient care and outcomes in PPH.

Q2. What is the impact of competency-based training on the knowledge and skills of health workers in management of postpartum hemorrhage?

Draft recommendations: Competency based training improves knowledge and skills in management of postpartum hemorrhage amongst all professional groups.

Evidence summary: In service training is a common method to address lack of skills amongst the health care providers to strengthen their knowledge, skills and attitudes. It is observed that multifaced interventions are better than single interventions and these should be succeeded by structured follow up interventions.

A structured optimum duration (2-3 weeks) of competency-based training including pretest assessment, theoretical lessons based on standard guidelines, followed by supervised frequent repetitive practice drills/ simulations (6–8 weeks, 30–40 min per week) based on clinical scenario using 'Low dose High Frequency Technique' should be undertaken in high priority areas. This is to be followed by post training assessment of skills using validated Objective Structured Clinical Examination (OSCE Checklist).

A recent cluster randomized trial to assess the effect of the training on knowledge and skills of health worker noted significant improvement in knowledge and skill s of health workers following one day training followed weekly practice drills for 6-8 weeks and high retention at 10 months follow up.

Another review of trainings for maternal and newborn health summarized that knowledge, skills and confidence of health care workers, clinical practices generally improves following such training, however, health outcomes vary, some studies showing improvement while others reported no effect following such training.

Two reviews noted a decrease in knowledge and skills 6-12 months after training, but the decrease did not reach the levels found before training.

Research gap: Research is needed to assess the decline in knowledge and skill levels after training to help facility management and policy makers plan for strategies to sustain skills and performance of available health workers.

Q3. What is the impact of Obstetric simulation and teamwork training on postpartum hemorrhage rates and outcomes.

Draft recommendations: Regular annual obstetric simulation and teamwork training significantly improves PPH Care and outcomes by timely well coordinated and systematic use of medical and refractory interventions there by reducing maternal morbidity, need for blood transfusion and surgical interventions.

Evidence summary: For effective implementation of PPH Safety bundles it is imperative that perinatal team members participate in regular annual simulation drills related to PPH. Obstetrics simulation and teamwork training provides realistic training, allows for sustainment of skills and prepares interdisciplinary team to respond more effectively to unpredictable challenges during emergencies.

A recent systematic review and meta-analysis on effect of obstetric emergency training on patient outcomes noted that effect of simulations PPH were unclear. However, in-situ multi-professional simulation training had the best impact in reducing the blood loss due to PPH and need for blood transfusion.

A recent Cochrane review noted that simulation based training in obstetric emergency may improve team performance and can lead to improved outcomes compared with no training however there is lack of high certainty evidence.

Similarly a prospective study on effect of obstetric simulation training on PPH rates and outcomes reported that though PPH rates did not change significantly, composite maternal morbidity, massive transfusion and mean postpartum length of stay decreased significantly while use of uterotonics and tranexamic acid and rate of surgical intervention decreased significantly.

Research gap: Need to assess the optimal frequency of training to support sustained improvement in PPH management.

Q4. What are the specific barriers faced by low resource settings in implementing FOGSI PPH EER?

Draft recommendations: Low resource settings face unique structural and functional barrier which contribute to high PPH mortality estimates.

Consequently PPH prevention and management in these settings require effective intervention tailored to the diverse needs of women and providers.

As part of efforts to implement this recommendation, health system stakeholders may consider the following potential barriers to their application:

- 50% or more of deliveries are attended by unskilled providers at home.
- Shortage of staff with the required expertise and skills to implement, supervise and support recommended practices.
- Lack of understanding of changes in recommended interventions among skilled care personnel and systems managers and resistance to changing from the use of non-evidence-based to evidence-based practices.
- Shortage of infrastructure to support interventions (such as power supply and refrigeration for storing oxytocin);
- Shortage of necessary equipment, drugs and consumables (such as needles, syringes, gloves and uterotonics);
- Absence of effective mechanisms to identify women who are experiencing PPH, in order to trigger PPH management pathways; and
- Ineffective health information management systems with improper documentation and monitoring (such as patient records and registers).

Q5. What strategies can be used to combat challenges in implementation and training of FOGSI PPH–EER in low resource settings.

Draft recommendations: Ensuring the existence and implementation of evidence based clinical guidelines is a key objective for prevention and management of PPH. An enabling environment should be created for the implementation of EER PPH recommendations, including education to support behavior change among skilled health personnel to facilitate the use of evidence-based practices.

Evidence summary: A systematic review studied the impact of implementation of updated guidelines for PPH management in clinical practice. Total seven trials were included. Out of these four trials reported decline in PPH cases after intervention. Another trial in Kazakhstan reported positive effect on PPH diagnosis and management when the guidelines when there was strict adherence to the guidelines. The evidence suggested that adherence to guidelines led to a more deliberated approach to the treatment of PPH.

Health care providers lack of awareness, lack of understanding of changes and resistance to changes from use of nonevidence based to evidence based practice are some of the key challenges.

Another Systematic meta-analysis concluded use of one single strategy is less effective for implementation of clinical guidelines as compared to strategy having multiple components.

National health systems need to ensure that availability of good-quality uterotonics and the necessary equipment in the facility providing maternity services. This will need establishing robust and sustainable regulatory, procurement and effective cold chain, and logistics processes.

Procurement agencies at all levels of supply chains should procure only quality-assured uterotonic medicines, that are labeled for storage at 2–8 °C, in single-use ampoules.

Use of uterine balloon tamponade will need appropriate training for skilled health personnel. Competency-based training, onsite, with training models and PPH emergency drills/simulations is advised, with periodic refresher training.

Administration of uterotonics currently requires the assistance of a skilled birth attendant (SBA), and therefore is not available to women experiencing unattended home births. WHO 2012 & GoI 2015 advocates for the distribution of misoprostol by lay health workers for home births. A double blind Randomized placebo controlled trial from Afghanistan testing a home based model care using misoprostol for prevention and treatment of Postpartum hemorrhage found Hb outcomes similar between the study groups (misoprostol: 56.4% (22/39), placebo: 60.6% (20/33), $p=0.45$). More women experienced shivering in misoprostol group (82.5% vs. placebo: 61.5%, $p=0.03$).

Another RCT using 800 µg of sublingual misoprostol to prevent and treat postpartum hemorrhage (PPH) during home delivery found no significant difference in clinical outcomes between the two trial arms

Strategies to combat challenges in training: Implementation of structured telementoring services seems to be a promising strategy to strengthen the technical and nontechnical competencies of the medical team in remote areas.

A systematic review noted that telementoring is effective in changing surgeons' knowledge and competence in both educational and workplace-based settings. Its use is also associated with changes in patient outcomes.

A recent mixed method study in Peru noted that implementation of telementoring program to provide guidance was a useful strategy for recently graduated medical professionals. However its use was limited due to connectivity issues, lack of anonymization when asking questions, and the presence of medical specialist mentors with whom they did not trust to ask openly.

Video based coaching is another alternative when telementoring is difficult to implement.

Q6. How can virtual and augmented Reality (AR &VR) tools be utilized to enhance training effectiveness for PPH management.

Draft recommendations: AR and VR tools have the potential to enhance the knowledge and skills of the students and improve their self-rated confidence levels by creating safe learning environment. It is suggested that this technology may function as an alternative to simulated clinical environment.

AR and VR represent two significant advances in immersive technology. AR overlays digital information into real world enhancing one 's perception of reality. It superimposes sounds, images or text on to our view of the real world scenario, providing interactive experiences and enabling us to visualize complex concepts in a real world context.

Virtual reality is a fully immersive experience where the user is placed with in a simulated environment. This technology allows us to interact with the digital environment as though it were real.

AR and VR have revolutionized the medical training remarkably. They offer a modern approach to patient consultations, surgical training, disease modeling and patient education.

Medical professionals who have used these technologies report improved understanding, increased confidence and patient outcomes. Also these technologies enable real time feedback helping learners understand their mistakes and correct them immediately. This enhances learning process, aids in the progressive improvement of the learners performance and enable the trainer to be psychologically prepared for high stress situations.

Summary of evidence: A two center two stage cross RCT comparing the satisfaction and effectiveness of virtual simulation with usual supervised work in producing knowledge and satisfaction amongst student midwives noted significantly higher satisfaction for the virtual simulation for its overall grade (6.8 vs. 6.1, $p = 0.009$) without lowering knowledge score

Another RCT investigated the use of a virtual reality learning environment (VRLE) to enhance medical student knowledge of postpartum hemorrhage (PPH) emergency management and insertion of a postpartum balloon noted VR may be beneficial in teaching hands-on procedural skills in obstetrics and gynecology education as it results in faster and enjoyable learning experience learning compared to traditional didactic learning.

Research gap: There is a need to analyze the cost effectiveness of the cost effectiveness of virtual reality teaching compared with traditional teaching.

BIBLIOGRAPHY

1. Abbas DF, Jehan N, Diop A, et al. Using misoprostol to treat postpartum hemorrhage in home deliveries attended by traditional birth attendants. Int J Gynaecol Obstet. 2019;144(3):290-6.
2. Abbas DF, Mirzazada S, Durocher J, et al. Testing a home-based model of care using misoprostol for prevention and treatment of postpartum hemorrhage: results from a randomized placebo-controlled trial conducted in Badakhshan province, Afghanistan. Reprod Health. 2020;17(1):88.

3. Alwy Al-beity F, Pembe AB, Marrone G, et al. Predictors of change of health c) workers' knowledge and skills after the Helping Mothers Survive Bleeding after Birth (HMS BAB) in-facility training in Tanzania. PLoS One. 2020;15(5):e0232983.
4. Ameh CA, Kerr R, Madaj B, et al. Knowledge and Skills of Healthcare Providers in Sub-Saharan Africa and Asia before and after Competency-Based Training in Emergency Obstetric and Early Newborn Care. PLos One. 2016;11(12): e0167270.
5. Bang A, Patel A, Bellad R, et al. Helping Babies Breathe (HBB) training: What happens to knowledge and skills over time? BMC pregnancy and childbirth. 2016;16(1):364. 9.
6. Brogaard L, Lauridsen KG, Lofgren B, et al. The effects of obstetric emergency team training on patient outcome: a systematic review and meta-analysis. Acta Obstet Gynecol Scand. 2022;101(1):25-36.
7. Dunlop K, Dillon G, McEvoy A, et al. The virtual reality classroom: a randomized control trial of medical student knowledge of postpartum hemorrhage emergency management. Front. Med. 2024;11:1371075.
8. Escobar M, Nassar AH, Theron G, et al. FIGO recommendations on the management of postpartum hemorrhage 2022. Int J Gynaecol Obstet. 2022;157 (Suppl 1): 3-50.
9. Fernandes RD, Ghasroddashti A, Sorefan-Mangou F, et al. Educational Effectiveness of Telementoring as a Continuing Professional Development Intervention for Surgeons in Practice: A Systematic Review. Ann Surg Open. 2023;4(4):e341.
10. Francke AL, Smit MC, de Veer AJ, et al. Factors influencing the implementation of clinical guidelines for health care professionals: A systematic meta-review. BMC Med Inform Decis Mak. 2008;8:38.
11. Fransen AF, van de Ven J, Banga FR, et al. Multi-professional simulation-based team training in obstetric emergencies for improving patient outcomes and trainees' performance. Cochrane Database Syst Re. 2020;12(12):CD011545.
12. Guidance note on Prevention and Management of Postpartum haemorrhage. India: Ministry Of Health and Family Welfare; 2015.
13. Lutgendorf MA, Ennen CS, McGlynn A, et al. Interprofessional obstetric simulation training improves postpartum haemorrhage management and decreases maternal morbidity: a before-and-after study. BJOG. 2024;131(3): 353-61.
14. Nadisauskiene RJ, Dobozinskas P, Kacerauskiene J, et al. The impact of the implementation of the postpartum haemorrhage management guidelines at the first regional perinatal centre in Southern Kazakhstan. BMC Pregnancy and Childbirth. 2016;16:238.
15. Nadisauskiene RJ, Kliucinskas M, Dobozinskas P, et al. The impact of postpartum haemorrhage management guidelines implemented in clinical practice: A systematic review of the literature. Eur J Obstet Gynecol Reprod Biol. 2014;178:21-26.
16. Nelissen E, Ersdal H, Mduma E, et al. Clinical performance and patient outcome after simulation-based training in prevention and management of postpartum haemorrhage: an educational intervention study in a low-resource setting. BMC Pregnancy and Childbirth. 2017;17(1):301.

17. Rojas-Mezarina L, Escobar-Agreda S, Chahuara-Rojas M, et al. Usability and perceptions of a one-on-one telementoring program for young physicians in rural settings of Peru: a mixed method study. BMC Med Educ. 2023; 23(1):175.
18. Rowe AK, Rowe SY, Peters DH, et al. Effectiveness of strategies to improve health-care provider practices in low-income and middle-income countries: a systematic review. The Lancet Global Health. 2018;6(11):e1163-e75.
19. Training Manual on PPH management–PPH Module-National Technical Committee on confidential enquiries into maternal deaths. India: Ministry of Family Welfare; 2016.
20. Van den Broek N, Ameh C, Madaj B, et al. Effects of emergency obstetric care training on maternal and perinatal outcomes: a stepped wedge cluster randomised trial in South Africa. BMJ Global Health. 2019; 4(6):e001670.
21. Voillequin S, Rozenberg P, Letutour K, et al. Comparative satisfaction and effectiveness of virtual simulation and usual supervised work for postpartum hemorrhage management: a crossover randomized controlled trial. BMC Med Educ. 2022;22(1):709.
22. WHO. Framework for action on interprofessional education and collaborative practice. Geneva: World Health Organization; 2010.
23. WHO. WHO recommendation on routes of oxytocin administration for the prevention of postpartum haemorrhage after vaginal birth. Geneva: World Health Organization; 2020.
24. WHO. WHO recommendation on uterine balloon tamponade for the treatment of postpartum haemorrhage. Geneva: World Health Organization; 2021.
25. WHO. WHO recommendations for the prevention and treatment of postpartum haemorrhage. Geneva: World Health Organization; 2012.
26. WHO. WHO recommendations on the assessment of postpartum blood loss and treatment bundles for postpartum haemorrhage. Geneva: World Health Organization; 2023.
27. Yang CW, Yen ZS, McGowan JE, et al. A systematic review of retention of adult advanced life support knowledge and skills in healthcare providers. Resuscitation. 2012;83(9):1055-60.

CHAPTER 15

Future More Trials Proposed for Indian Innovations

Mahesh Gupta, Manish R Pandya

We proudly say that there are few innovators in India who had worked very hard to develop and propose the means to control postpartum hemorrhage (PPH).

Namely:

1. *Mechanical means of controlling the PPH*
   a. *Chhattisgarh condom tamponade (CG Balloon by Nalini Mishra and team):* Separate chapter about minimal surgical management mentioning the device is written in this book (Chapter 8). It is not a commercial device but is easily prepared at the point of care. This modified condom balloon tamponade device can be prepared in advance and kept ready to use by getting it through the process of ETO. It has a central drainage port to assess the ongoing blood loss in real time. It also enables the vagina to be packed before inflation of the balloon which prevents its expulsion during the process of inflation. This device has been mentioned in FIGO recommendations for management of PPH 2022. It was also considered to be one of the most cost effective options in a systematic review of cost-effectiveness of uterine tamponade devices for the treatment of postpartum hemorrhage. There are observational studies to support Condom Tamponade, we request our FOGSIAN to work on it and publish their cases to make a more strong evidences. It is to be kept ready in all cases of Atonic PPH after Normal labor. It may also be used in refractory PPH after caesarean section.
   b. *Vacuum suction devices (SR Canula and Panikar Canula by Samarth Ram and TN Vasudeva Panikar):* It is also observed that there are few studies to support the use of various vacuum devices to use during PPH. Indian vacuum suction device is also getting popular, so it has also become a choice for atonic PPH after normal labor. It may also be used in refractory PPH after caesarean section. All FOGSIAN are requested to publish their experience to show the effectiveness.
   c. *COMOC MG (Compression of myometrium and occlusion of uterine artery—Mahesh Gupta):* It is an Indian surgical means of tackling the

atonic PPH, where special suture is also available in suture market. It is an easy, quick, and reproducible to perform. The advantage of being one puncture on one side, one can perform two modalities of the PPH tackling surgery, that vertical compression of myometrium and occlusion of uterine vessels **(Figs. 1A to F)**.

This technique will give very promising results if perform early.

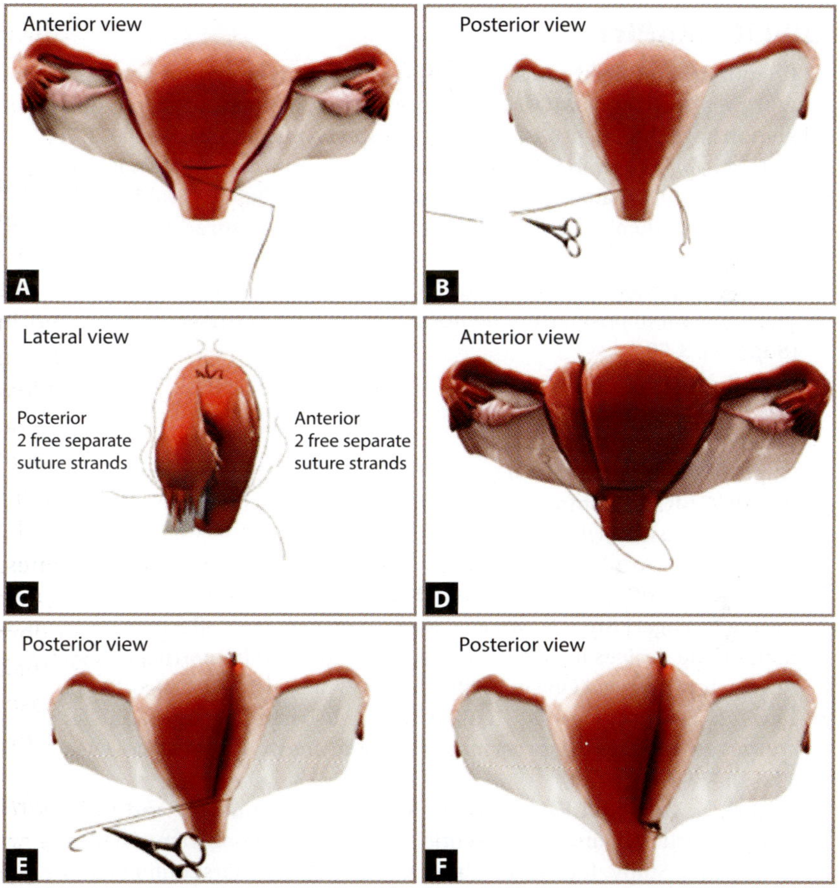

Figs. 1A to F: COMOC-MG Stitch. Notes: (A) 80-mm long straight taper point needle is inserted into the uterus from 3 cm below and 3 cm medial to the lower cut edge of the uterus; (B) The loop around the eye of the needle is cut to obtain two free limbs posteriorly and two free limbs anteriorly; (C) From double strand, one strand will make a loop on the top of uterus as Hayman's suture; (D) The second strand with round body needle will now pass to the avascular area just below the cut edge of uterus at the same level on the posterior aspect and (E and F) both limbs of the second suture strand tied firmly to occlude the uterine artery.

Till date more than 120 cases are published and also published as a technique in Springer journal.

RCOG also endorsed this technique.

Few dissertations also done in various medical college.

Even in Spain, it has been translated in Spanish language and presented in Spain conference.

It is available in YouTube also and readymade suture material is available in Indian market.

BIBLIOGRAPHY

1. Chaudhari TJ. Effectiveness of compression of myometrium and occlusion of uterine artery by COMOC-MG suture in management of atonic postpartum hemorrhage. Int J Reprod Contracept Obstet Gynecol. 2024;13(4):971-7.
2. Damor P, Maheshwari S, Singh S. Role of SR vacuum cannula as novel technique for atonic PPH management study at Pannadhay Rajkiya Mahila Chikitsalaya and RNT Medical College, Udaipur. Int J Reprod Contracept Obstet Gynecol 2021;10:4150-6.
3. Escobar M, Nassar AH, Theron G, et al. FIGO recommendations on the management of postpartum hemorrhage 2022. Int J Gynaecol Obstet. 2022;157 (Suppl 1): 3-50.
4. Garg R, Yadav A. Condom Balloon Tamponade for Postpartum Hemorrhage in Developing Countries: Cost-effective Boon for Saving Mothers. J South Asian Feder Obst Gyne. 2022;14(2):189-91.
5. Gupta M, Gupta A, Otha DD, et al. Modification of B-Lynch Stitch Technique (COMOC MG) to Control Postpartum Hemorrhage: Clinical Perspective from 19 Cases. Pan Asian J Obs Gyn. 2020;3(2):98-102.
6. Hayman RG, Arulkumaran S, Steer PJ. Uterine compression sutures: surgical management of postpartum hemorrhage. Obstet Gynecol. 2002;99(3): 502-6.
7. Joshua P. Vogel | Alyce N. Wilson | Nick Scott et al. Cost-effectiveness of uterine tamponade devices for the treatment of postpartum hemorrhage: A systematic review. Int J Gynecol Obstet 2020; 151: 333–340 DOI:10.1002/ijgo.13393.
8. Kaveh M, Tahermanesh K, Hanjani S, et al. B-lynch plus technique for uterine conservative surgery in an asymmetric atonic uterus. Int J Gynecol Obstet. 2018; 142(3):370-1.
9. Mishra N, Gulabani K, Agrawal S, Shrivastava S. Efficacy and Feasibility of Chhattisgarh Balloon and Conventional Condom Balloon Tamponade: A 2-Year Prospective Study. Journal of Obstet Gynaecol India. First online Jan 5: (2019); 1-9. https://doi.org/10.1007/s13224-018-1185-6.
10. Mishra N, Shrivastava C, Agrawal S, Gulabani K. The CG balloon is an innovative condom balloon tamponade for the management of postpartum hemorrhage in low-resource settings. International Journal of Gynecology and Obstetrics (2016). http://dx.doi.org/10.1016/j.ijgo.2015.10.014.
11. Mishra N, Shrivastava C, Agrawal S. et al. Easy Balloon: The Easiest to Assemble Condom Balloon Uterine Tamponade for Primary Level of Health Care Centres. J Obstet Gynecol India Oct. 2017; 67(5):378-81. doi:10.1007/s13224-017-1014-3.

12. Moleiro ML, Braga J, Machado MJ, et al. Uterine compression sutures in controlling postpartum haemorrhage: a narrative review. Acta Méd Port. 2022; 35(1):51-8.
13. Montgomery AL, Ram U, Kumar R, et al. Maternal mortality in India: causes and healthcare service use based on a nationally representative survey. PLoS One. 2014;9(1):e83331.
14. Prajapati J, Oza A, Gupta M, et al. The compression of myometrium and occlusion of uterine artery by COMOC-MG technique for the management of postpartum haemorrhage: clinical perspective from ten cases. Int J Reprod Contracept Obstet Gynecol. 2024;13:1020.
15. Rana V, Patel A, Patel V. Use of Panicker's cannula in management of atonic postpartum hemorrhage. Int J Reprod Contracept Obstet Gynecol. 2024;13: 1277-80.
16. Zahid. (2017). Postpartum haemorrhage. [online] Available from https://www.nhp.gov.in/disease/gynaecology-and-obstetrics/postpartum-haemorrhage. [Last accessed November, 2024].

Summary

Sheela Mane

Postpartum hemorrhage (PPH) represents a significant global health challenge, constituting a leading cause of maternal morbidity and mortality. Despite advancements in obstetric care, PPH continues to disproportionately affect women in low- and middle-income countries. The condition is characterized by excessive blood loss following childbirth, often resulting in severe complications including hypovolemic shock, organ dysfunction, and death. Comprehensive prevention and management strategies are essential to reduce the burden of PPH and improve maternal outcomes worldwide.

Standardization of terminology and diagnostic criteria for postpartum hemorrhage (PPH) is essential for accurate clinical assessment, research, and quality improvement. Currently, a lack of consensus exists regarding PPH definitions and severity grading, hindering data comparability, and clinical decision-making. While blood loss quantification is valuable, hemodynamic instability, as reflected by changes in vital signs, is a more reliable indicator of PPH severity. The development of standardized tools for assessing blood loss and clinical status is crucial to improve early identification and management of PPH.

While various risk factors have been identified, it is important to note that over half of PPH cases occur without identifiable risk factors. Risk factors for PPH can be categorized into antepartum and intrapartum factors. Common risk factors include previous history of PPH, uterine fibroids, multiple pregnancies, preeclampsia, and prolonged labor. These factors often contribute to the four main causes of PPH: uterine atony (weakness of the uterus), trauma (lacerations), retained placental tissue, and coagulopathy (blood clotting disorders). Risk assessment tools, such as the CMQCC, ACOG SMI, and AWOHNN, can help identify women at increased risk of PPH. However, these tools have limitations in predicting severe PPH and should be used in conjunction with clinical judgment. Recent studies suggest an increasing incidence of PPH, potentially due to factors like rising cesarean section rates, obesity, and induction of labor. Additionally, risk factors may vary across different ethnic groups, highlighting the need for culturally sensitive care.

Prevention of PPH is critical to maternal health. Effective strategies encompass antenatal care to manage risk factors such as anemia and preeclampsia. During labor, judicious use of induction and augmentation is essential, while active management of the third stage of labor, including uterotonic administration, is paramount. Addressing the specific needs of resource-limited settings, with a focus on community-based interventions and task shifting, is crucial. Continued research on emerging technologies and the refinement of prevention strategies are necessary to further optimize maternal outcomes.

Remember the Golden hour—Quick and efficient management is extremely important to avoid mortality and morbidity. Effective PPH management requires rapid diagnosis, a multidisciplinary team, and immediate action. Early identification and classification of PPH severity are crucial. Prompt resuscitation, including airway, breathing, circulation, disability, and exposure (ABCDE) assessment, is essential. Simultaneously, the cause of bleeding must be determined and addressed. A combination of uterotonic medications, fluid resuscitation, blood products, and potentially surgical interventions may be necessary. In resource-limited settings, focus is on early recognition, available uterotonics, and efficient transfer to higher-level care. Continuous research is needed to improve PPH management and outcomes.

Prophylactic measures to mitigate postpartum hemorrhage (PPH) include early identification and treatment of anemia, judicious use of anticoagulants, implementation of active management of the third stage of labor, and meticulous surgical technique. Blood transfusion is indicated in PPH when hemodynamic instability, characterized by tachycardia and hypotension, manifests despite conservative measures. Blood transfusion necessitates informed consent; however, in life-threatening emergencies, immediate transfusion may precede formal consent acquisition. Selection of blood components, including packed red blood cells, fresh frozen plasma, platelets, cryoprecipitate, fibrinogen concentrate, and, in specific circumstances, recombinant Factor VIIa and prothrombin complex concentrate, is essential for optimal resuscitation. For severe hemorrhage, a massive transfusion protocol is activated to expedite the delivery of blood products. Vigilant monitoring for transfusion reactions is crucial. Thus, the judicious use of blood components, complemented by advanced monitoring tools and protocols, is paramount in optimizing maternal outcomes.

Refractory postpartum hemorrhage (PPH) is a severe obstetric complication characterized by persistent, excessive blood loss despite initial management efforts. This condition is often associated with hemodynamic instability. Effective management necessitates a comprehensive approach, including prompt recognition, aggressive resuscitation, and a stepwise implementation of therapeutic interventions. Key strategies encompass addressing the underlying etiology, uterotonic administration, and a combination of mechanical maneuvers such as aortic compression, uterine massage, and uterine balloon tamponade. In refractory cases, invasive procedures like selective arterial embolization may be considered.

Pelvic vasculature ligation is a critical component of the surgical management of refractory PPH, but it should be performed by experienced surgeons in appropriate clinical settings.

Emergency peripartum hysterectomy (EPH) is a life-saving procedure performed to control severe, uncontrollable postpartum hemorrhage (PPH) that does not respond to other treatments. Factors like uterine atony, placental abnormalities, and uterine rupture often necessitate EPH. Despite its effectiveness, it carries significant risks and impacts women's fertility. Efforts are focused on preventing PPH and developing alternative treatments to reduce the need for hysterectomy.

Certain patient groups have an elevated risk of postpartum hemorrhage (PPH). Women with multiple pregnancies, severe preeclampsia, obesity, and those with uterine fibroids are more likely to experience PPH compared to the general population. While aspirin use for preeclampsia prevention generally does not increase PPH risk, discontinuation prior to delivery is recommended. Intrahepatic cholestasis of pregnancy does not appear to influence PPH risk. Early intervention and specific management strategies are crucial for these high-risk groups. Key preventive measures include the use of carbetocin over oxytocin in severe preeclampsia and obesity, and maintaining heightened awareness for PPH in all identified risk groups.

To effectively combat postpartum hemorrhage (PPH), a multi-pronged approach is needed. This includes equipping healthcare providers with detection tools, training programs, and clear communication methods. Regular evaluations and community outreach programs further strengthen this strategy. By integrating digital health applications and simulation training, healthcare facilities can significantly improve their ability to manage PPH, leading to better maternal health outcomes.

A structured training and implementation play an important role in effective PPH management. This includes developing comprehensive training modules, identifying skilled trainers, and establishing appropriate training durations. Competency-based training, simulation exercises, and teamwork drills are crucial for enhancing healthcare provider skills. Addressing challenges in low-resource settings, such as infrastructure limitations and staff shortages, is essential. Leveraging technology, including tele-mentoring and virtual reality, can further improve training effectiveness.

By standardizing care, promoting early intervention, and addressing specific risk factors, these guidelines aim to improve maternal outcomes globally. This document is designed for healthcare providers across various settings, from resource-rich hospitals to community clinics. By implementing these recommendations, healthcare facilities can significantly enhance their capacity to prevent and manage PPH, ultimately reducing maternal morbidity and mortality.

